PHYSICIAN
ASSISTANT

EXAMINATION REVIEW

PHYSICIAN
ASSISTANT

SECOND EDITION

850
Multiple-choice Questions with
Explanatory Answers

Richard R. Rahr, EdD, PA-C
Chairman and Professor

Bruce R. Niebuhr, PhD
Associate Professor

*Department of Physician's
Assistant Studies
School of Allied Health Sciences
The University of Texas Medical
Branch
Galveston, Texas*

MEDICAL EXAMINATION PUBLISHING COMPANY

Notice: The author(s) and the publisher of this volume have taken care that the information and recommendations contained herein are accurate and compatible with the standards generally accepted at the time of publication. Nevertheless, it is difficult to ensure that all the information given is entirely accurate for all circumstances. The publisher disclaims any liability, loss, or damage incurred as a consequence, directly or indirectly, of the use and application of any of the contents of this volume.

94 95 96 97 / 10 9 8 7 6 5 4 3 2

Prentice Hall International (UK) Limited, *London*
Prentice Hall of Australia Pty. Limited, *Sydney*
Prentice Hall Canada, Inc., *Toronto*
Prentice Hall Hispanoamericana, S.A., *Mexico*
Prentice Hall of India Private Limited, *New Delhi*
Prentice Hall of Japan, Inc., *Tokyo*
Simon & Schuster Asia Pte. Ltd., *Singapore*
Editora Prentice Hall do Brasil Ltda., *Rio de Janeiro*
Prentice Hall, *Englewood Cliffs, New Jersey*

ISBN 0-8385-8026-2

Library of Congress Catalog Card Number: 92-083805

PRINTED IN THE UNITED STATES OF AMERICA

Contents

Preface

Physician Assistant Examination Review, Second Edition, is designed to aid individuals in preparing for the certifying examination administered by the National Commission on Certification of Physician Assistants. The book contains multiple-choice questions in formats similar to those used in the certifying examination. A wide range of medical and surgical topics are covered.

The questions in this book have been prepared by a group of leading physician assistant educators to encompass the depth and breadth of medical knowledge and practice as it relates to the physician assistant. We wish to thank the contributors to this book for providing such excellent questions.

Richard R. Rahr
Bruce R. Niebuhr
Galveston, Texas

Contributors

J. Dennis Blessing, PhD, PA-C, Department of Physician Assistant Studies, The University of Texas Medical Branch, Galveston, Texas

Collier M. Cole, PhD, Department of Physician Assistant Studies, The University of Texas Medical Branch, Galveston, Texas

William R. Duryea, PhD, PA-C, Physician Assistant Program, St. Francis College, Loretto, Pennsylvania

Carl E. Fasser, PA-C, Physician Assistant Program, Baylor College of Medicine, Houston, Texas

John Fuchs, Jr, PharmD, Pharmacy Department, The University of Texas Medical Branch, Galveston, Texas

Elaine E. Grant, PA-C, Physician Associate Program, Yale University School of Medicine, New Haven, Connecticut

Gary C. Johnson, MEd, PA-C, Physician Assistant Program, Trevecca Nazarene College, Nashville, Tennessee

Barbara Ann Lyons, MA, PA-C, Department of Physician Assistant Studies, The University of Texas Medical Branch, Galveston, Texas

Richard D. Muma, PA-C, Department of Physician Assistant Studies, The University of Texas Medical Branch, Galveston, Texas

Richard Rivera, MS, PA-C, Department of Physician Assistant Studies, The University of Texas Medical Branch, Galveston, Texas

Jan Victoria Scott, MHS, PA-C, Physician Assistant Program, Duke University Medical Center, Durham, North Carolina

Steven R. Shelton, MBA, PA-C, Department of Physician Assistant Studies, The University of Texas Medical Branch, Galveston, Texas

Karen S. Stephenson, PA-C, Department of Physician Assistant Studies, The University of Texas Medical Branch, Galveston, Texas

Laura J. Stuetzer, MS, PA-C, Department of Physician Assistant Education, St. Louis University Medical Center, St. Louis, Missouri

Janice V. Tramel, PA-C, Primary Care Physician Assistant Program, University of Southern California, School of Medicine, Los Angeles, California

1 Genitourinary System

DIRECTIONS (Questions 1–35): Each of the questions or incomplete statements below is followed by four or five suggested answers or completions. Select the **one** that is best in each case.

1. MOST noncomplicated, nonnosocomial urinary tract infections are caused by
    A. *Escherichia coli*
    B. *Chlamydia trachomatis*
    C. *Neisseria gonorrhoeae*
    D. *Pseudomonas aeruginosa*
    E. *Gardnerella vaginalis*

2. Which of the following is **NOT** a sign or symptom of acute cystitis?
    A. Dysuria
    B. Suprapubic pain
    C. Urgency
    D. Flank pain
    E. Nocturia

3. Which of the following is **NOT** indicated in the evaluation of acute bacterial prostatitis?
    A. Rectal examination
    B. Urinalysis
    C. Transurethral instrumentation
    D. CBC
    E. Urine culture and sensitivity

4. In males, gonococcal urethritis
    A. is always symptomatic
    B. spontaneously resolves after three months
    C. presents with a scant, clear discharge
    D. is transmitted by vaginal intercourse only
    E. usually presents with urethral discharge and dysuria

5. *C. trachomatis*
    A. rarely causes epididymitis in men under 35 years old
    B. is always symptomatic
    C. is not a sexually transmitted disease
    D. is present in 80% of men with Reiter's syndrome
    E. is a gram-negative, intracellular diplococcus

6. Renal calculi are **MOST** commonly
    A. uric acid
    B. calcium oxalate
    C. calcium phosphate
    D. cystine
    E. a combination of calcium oxalate and phosphate

7. The common sites of renal stone impaction include all of the following **EXCEPT**
    A. the ureteropelvic junction
    B. the ureterovesical junction
    C. the level of crossing of the ureter over the iliac vessels
    D. the vesicourethral junction

8. Which of the following findings on IVP indicates the need for immediate referral to a urologist for a patient with renal colic?
   A. Bilateral renal calculi
   B. Prompt excretion of dye by both kidneys
   C. Nonobstructing ureteral stone
   D. Unilateral total obstruction of ureter
   E. Bladder stone

9. A thin clear discharge that continues following penicillin treatment of gonococcal urethritis is **MOST** likely due to
   A. inadequate treatment
   B. a resistant strain of *N. gonorrhoeae*
   C. urethral inflammation
   D. benign posttreatment discharge
   E. concurrent infection by *C. trachomatis*

10. The single most useful **SCREENING** test for GU disease is
    A. urinalysis
    B. CBC
    C. 24-hour urine
    D. BUN
    E. creatinine

11. A contraindication to catheterization in the management of acutely injured patients is
    A. pelvic injury
    B. abdominal injury
    C. spinal fracture
    D. blood in the urethral meatus
    E. shock

12. Which of the following is **NOT** consistent with nephrotic syndrome?
    A. Massive edema
    B. Less than one gram proteinuria in 24-hour urine
    C. Hypoalbuminemia
    D. Hyperlipidemia
    E. Anemia

13. The **MOST** common sign of a genitourinary tract tumor is
   A. pain
   B. dysuria
   C. hematuria
   D. palpable mass

14. Nephroblastoma (Wilms' tumor) is a malignant renal tumor that occurs primarily in
   A. males
   B. females
   C. blacks
   D. whites
   E. children

15. The **MOST** common tumor of the GU tract is cancer of the
   A. urethra
   B. prostate
   C. bladder
   D. ureter
   E. kidney

16. Which of the following is **NOT** true of prostate cancer?
   A. It is rarely diagnosed in men under 50 years of age
   B. Common metastatic sites are the spine and pelvis
   C. Soft, indiscreet, symmetrical nodules usually are cancerous
   D. Obstructive symptoms are common

17. Which of the following should increase suspicion of prostatic cancer?
   A. Rapid onset and progression of symptoms
   B. Incomplete emptying of bladder and pain
   C. Hesitancy, dribbling, and urgency
   D. Loss of force and decreased caliber of stream

18. Malignancy of the testis
   A. is relatively common
   B. is directly related to testicular trauma
   C. generally presents as a painful mass
   D. occurs primarily in younger men
   E. has a very poor prognosis

19. Which of the following is a useful marker for prostatic cancer?
   A. Testosterone
   B. Acid phosphatase
   C. Alkaline phosphatase
   D. Parathyroid hormone

20. Which is **NOT** true of prostate-specific antigen (PSA) in prostate cancer?
   A. It is elevated in 100% of prostate cancer cases
   B. It returns to normal quickly following effective treatment
   C. It increases early in recurrence
   D. It can be elevated in BPH

21. Which is **TRUE** of men with varicocele?
   A. It never occurs in men less than 40 years old
   B. The right side is more commonly affected
   C. Infertility is a common, associated problem
   D. The patient must be examined in the supine position

22. Torsion of the testis
   A. is always preceded by injury to the scrotum
   B. is always preceded by UTI
   C. is a surgical emergency
   D. usually affects men over 40 years of age
   E. is all of the above

23. Which is **NOT** a sign or symptom of acute pyelonephritis?
   A. Insidious onset
   B. Shaking chills, and fever
   C. Malaise, nausea, and vomiting
   D. Flank or back pain
   E. Symptoms of cystitis

24. The empirical treatment of acute pyelonephritis should include all of the following **EXCEPT**
   A. urine for culture and sensitivity studies
   B. hydration
   C. control of pain and fever
   D. bedrest
   E. antimicrobial treatment based on culture and sensitivity results

25. The recommended choices for empirical treatment of pyelone-phritis (provided there are no contraindications to the drug, such as allergy) are
    A. ampicillin and an aminoglycoside
    B. tetracycline and a cephalosporin
    C. ampicillin and a cephalosporin
    D. penicillin and tetracycline
    E. erythromycin and chloramphenicol

26. Curvature of the penis secondary to fibrous plaque of the penile shaft is
    A. priapism
    B. Peyronie's disease
    C. phimosis
    D. paraphimosis

27. Which is **NOT** true concerning circumcision?
    A. It is routinely performed for religious or cultural reasons
    B. It is indicated in patients with chronic infections, phimosis, or paraphimosis
    C. Uncircumcised men have a lower incidence of penile carcinoma
    D. Poor hygiene and chronic infection are underlying factors in penile carcinoma in uncircumcised men

28. Which of the following is **NOT** true of acute epididymitis?
    A. It may follow severe physical strain or considerable sexual excitement
    B. Onset of severe pain is sudden and the epididymis is exquisitely sensitive
    C. The scrotum is usually enlarged and the overlying skin is erythemic
    D. Swelling is insidious, slow, and difficult to detect early in the disease process
    E. The WBC is markedly elevated, with a shift to the left

29. Which of the following is **NOT** true of acute epididymitis?
    A. Complete resolution may take 2 to 4 weeks or more
    B. Complications are common
    C. Bedrest, scrotal support, ice packs, and analgesia are components of treatment
    D. Antibiotics are always part of the treatment process
    E. Fertility problems may occur, particularly if the process is bilateral

30. Which of the following is **TRUE** concerning acute pyelonephritis?
    A. It involves renal pelvis only
    B. It always affects both kidneys
    C. Infection by *E. coli* is rare
    D. It may involve the renal pelvis and parenchyma
    E. All of the above

31. Which of the following is **TRUE** concerning UTI?
    A. Ureteritis is a distinct type of UTI
    B. Ureteritis requires specific treatment
    C. Specific signs and symptoms are indicative of ureteritis
    D. Isolated infection of the ureter does not occur

32. Which of the following may be used to treat an uncomplicated cystitis in women?
    A. Sulfonamides
    B. Trimethoprim-sulfamethoxazole
    C. Nitrofurantoin
    D. Ampicillin/amoxicillin
    E. All of the above

33. The empirical drug of choice in the management of acute prostatitis is
    A. sulfonamide
    B. trimethoprim-sulfamethoxazole
    C. nitrofurantoin
    D. ampicillin/amoxicillin
    E. all of the above

34. Which of the following is **TRUE** concerning infertility?
   A. Any generalized fever or illness can impair spermatogenesis
   B. Most infertility problems are due to a female factor
   C. History and physical examination generally contribute little to the evaluation of male infertility
   D. Concurrent evaluation of both partners is unnecessary if one or the other is being evaluated
   E. All of the above are true

35. Which of the following is a treatment option for impotence?
   A. Prosthesis implant
   B. Vacuum and band device
   C. Injection of vasoactive drugs
   D. Counseling
   E. All of the above

Explanatory Answers

1. A. In acute infections, a single organism is usually found. *E. coli* is the most common infective agent. (Ref. 1, p. 196)

2. D. Flank pain is indicative of pyelonephritis, rather than cystitis. (Ref. 1, p. 221)

3. C. Transurethral instrumentation, including catheterization, should be avoided during the acute phase of prostatitis. (Ref. 1, p. 223)

4. E. Gonococcal urethritis in men usually presents with urethral discharge and dysuria. The discharge is usually yellow or brown. The disease may be asymptomatic in some patients. If untreated, the symptoms will resolve in 95% of patients in three months; however, the patient is not disease-free. GC may be transmitted by vaginal, rectal, or oral intercourse. (Ref. 1, p. 262)

5. D. *C. trachomatis* is the leading cause of epididymitis in men under age 35, may be asymptomatic, is sexually transmitted, and is present in the genital tract of 80% of men with Reiter's syndrome. It is a small bacterium and an obligate intracellular parasite of the epithelium. (Ref. 1, p. 267)

6. E. Calcium stones are most commonly a mixture of calcium oxalate and calcium phosphate. Calcium oxalate is the sole or major component in 80% of all stones. (Ref. 1, p. 279)

7. D. The three points of ureteral narrowing are the ureteropelvic junction, the point where the ureter crosses the iliac vessels, and the ureterovesical zone. (Ref. 1, p. 276)

8. D. Total obstruction of renal outflow can lead to hydronephrosis and renal parenchymal damage in a short period of time. (Ref. 1, p. 291)

9. E. Concurrent infection with *C. trachomatis* occurs in 10% to 35% of men with gonorrhea. (Ref. 1, p. 265)

10. A. A number of tests are available for evaluation of the renal and

GU systems. The urinalysis is most available as a screening tool. (Ref. 1, p. 46)

11. D.   Blood at the urethral meatus indicates urethral injury that needs to be evaluated prior to catheterization. (Ref. 1, p. 302)

12. B.   Heavy protein loss is a key to the diagnosis of nephrotic syndrome. The urine may contain 4 to 10 grams of protein per 24 hours. (Ref. 1, p. 518)

13. C.   Gross or microscopic hematuria is the most common sign of GU tumor. (Ref. 1, p. 330)

14. E.   Wilm's tumor occurs primarily in young children (median age 2 years, 11 months) without significant differentiation between males and females or race. (Ref. 1, p. 344)

15. B.   Prostate cancer is the most common neoplasm in men and of the GU tract. (Ref. 1, p. 366)

16. C.   Asymmetrical, hard, discrete nodules of the prostate have a greater than 50% chance of being cancerous. (Ref. 1, p. 370)

17. A.   Enlargement of the prostate produces obstructive symptoms, regardless of the cause, but rapid onset and progression is more ominous. (Ref. 1, p. 369)

18. D.   Primary tumors of the testes tend to occur in younger age groups. (Ref. 1, p. 385)

19. B.   Acid phosphatase is still a useful marker for prostatic cancer. Alkaline phosphatase is a useful marker for bone metastasis from prostate cancer. (Ref. 1, p. 55)

20. A.   PSA is elevated in approximately 60% of prostate cancer patients. (Ref. 1, p. 55)

21. C.   Varicocele is found in 10% of young men; 65% to 75% of patients have decreased sperm concentration; it occurs most commonly on the left; and examination is best performed with the patient standing. (Ref. 1, p. 593)

22. C.   Men of any age can have torsion of the testicle, but it is primarily a phenomenon of boys under the age of 16. There is usually no antecedent event, and immediate surgical exploration and correction is necessary. (Ref. 1, p. 595)

23. A.   The symptoms and signs of acute pyelonephritis usually begin abruptly. (Ref. 1, p. 202)

24. E.   Antibiotic therapy should be empirical until culture and sensitivity results are available. (Ref. 1, p. 204)

25. A.   Ampicillin and an aminoglycoside are a logical choice of antibiotics that cover the major pathogens known to cause pyelonephritis. (Ref. 1, p. 204)

26. B.   Dense, fibrous plaque of varying size and involving the tunica albuginea that may cause curvature of the penis, painful erections, and prevent vaginal penetration during attempted intercourse is Peyronie's disease. (Ref. 1, p. 575)

27. C.   Uncircumcised men have a higher incidence of penile carcinoma; but hygiene and chronic infection seem to be underlying factors. (Ref. 1, p. 576)

28. D.   Swelling is rapid and may cause the affected organ to double in size within 3 to 4 hours. (Ref. 1, p. 229)

29. B.   Complications are rare after prompt, appropriate treatment. (Ref. 1, p. 230)

30. D.   Acute pyelonephritis is an infectious inflammatory disease that involves both the renal parenchyma and pelvis of one or both kidneys. *E. coli* is the predominant pathogen. (Ref. 1, p. 201)

31. D.   Ureteritis may occur with other infections of the urinary tract, but is of little clinical importance. (Ref. 1, p. 220)

32. E.   Most uncomplicated, community acquired infections are due to *E. coli*; any of the drugs listed are effective. (Ref. 1, p. 221)

33. B.   Until culture and sensitivity results are known, and since the causative organisms are usually gram-negative rods, trimethoprim-sul-famethoxazole is a good choice. (Ref. 1, p. 224)

34. A. Problems in men and women contribute equally to couple infertility. Concurrent evaluation is recommended, with the history and physical examination being major components. (Ref. 1, p. 643)

35. E. All of the items listed are possible treatment forms for impotence. (Ref. 1, p. 669)

2 Pharmacology

DIRECTIONS (Questions 36–78): Each of the questions or incomplete statements below is followed by four or five suggested answers or completions. Select the **one** that is best in each case.

---

36. Drug effect is a result of interaction between the drug and
    A. cell receptors
    B. blood serum levels
    C. electrolyte balance
    D. the physical state of being

37. A drug that initiates a cell reaction is called
    A. an antagonist
    B. an agonist
    C. an active transporter
    D. a filtrator

38. A drug that inhibits or competes with a substance for a receptor is
    A. an antagonist
    B. an agonist
    C. an active transporter
    D. a filtrator

39. The measurement of drug disappearance is called the
   A. time-to-disappearance
   B. drug lifetime
   C. drug effect-time
   D. biological half-life

40. Which organ system is involved with drug excretion?
   A. Kidneys
   B. Lungs
   C. Liver
   D. Intestines
   E. All of the above

41. Which is **NOT** a renal factor in the urinary excretion of a drug?
   A. Glomerular filtration rate
   B. Extent of back diffusion
   C. Extent of active tubular secretion
   D. Extent of active tubular reabsorption
   E. Volume of drug distribution

42. Which of the following is **TRUE** concerning phase 1 drug studies?
   A. They are animal studies only
   B. They usually involve only very ill patients
   C. They must include women and children to be valid
   D. They are usually conducted on healthy males, aged 18 to 45

43. Which of the following is **TRUE** concerning phase 2 drug studies?
   A. First trials in ill patients
   B. Patients must have multiple, serious illnesses
   C. Minimum number of subjects is 1000
   D. Dose response is unimportant
   E. All of the above

44. Which of the following is **NOT** true concerning phase 3 drug studies?
   A. Large number of subjects
   B. Designed to verify efficacy
   C. Adverse reactions are unimportant
   D. Designed to detect effects not seen in phases 1 and 2
   E. Usually completed prior to drug release for use

45. Which of the following is **TRUE** of phase 4 drug studies?
   A. Always controlled studies
   B. Always uncontrolled studies
   C. Women, children, and older adults are excluded
   D. Allow for continued evaluation of a drug
   E. Last phase prior to release of drug to public

46. Heparin effect is monitored by
   A. prothrombin time (PT)
   B. partial thromboplastin time (PTT)
   C. white blood cell count (WBC)
   D. red blood cell count (RBC)

47. Adequate heparin therapy should raise the PTT to
   A. the mean laboratory value
   B. five times normal
   C. 50% below normal
   D. 3 to 4 times normal
   E. 1.5 to 2 times normal

48. Which of the following increases the anticoagulant effect of warfarin (Coumadin)?
   A. Rifampin
   B. Barbiturates
   C. Cholestyramine
   D. Salicylates
   E. Vitamin K (large doses)

49. The antibacterial action of penicillins and cephalosporins is
   A. inhibition of cell wall synthesis
   B. inhibition of protein synthesis
   C. interference with cell membrane function
   D. interference with DNA/RNA replication

50. Which of the following is bacteriostatic?
   A. Ampicillin
   B. Rifampin
   C. Bacitracin
   D. Tetracycline
   E. All of the above

51. The penicillins are generally effective against which of the following microorganisms?
  A. *S. pneumoniae*
  B. *H. influenzae*
  C. *N. gonorrhoeae*
  D. *E. coli*
  E. All of the above

52. Which of the following is **NOT** true concerning cephalosporins?
  A. Similar to the penicillins in structure
  B. Have a more narrow spectrum than penicillin G
  C. Greater degree of beta-lactamase stability than the penicillins
  D. Relatively nontoxic
  E. There is some cross-sensitivity in penicillin-allergic patients

53. When indicated, a suitable drug for penicillin-allergic patients is
  A. dicloxacillin
  B. nafcillin
  C. erythromycin
  D. ampicillin

54. Cimetidine (Tagamet) is
  A. an H_2 agonist
  B. contraindicated in Zollinger-Ellison syndrome
  C. given parenterally only
  D. used for active/prophylactic treatment of peptic ulcers

55. The role of probenecid in the treatment of gout is to
  A. increase plasma levels of uric acid
  B. increase uric acid deposition into joints
  C. potentiate the effect of NSAID and colchicine
  D. block active reabsorption of uric acid

56. Which antiasthmatic is **NOT** effective in acute episodes?
  A. Cromolyn sodium
  B. Epinephrine
  C. Terbutaline
  D. Theophylline

57. The initial drug of choice in the conservative treatment of rheumatoid arthritis is
   A. colchicine
   B. penicillamine
   C. prednisone
   D. acetaminophen
   E. aspirin

58. Sucralfate (Carafate), used in the treatment of peptic ulcers, is
   A. an H_2 antagonist
   B. an anticholinergic
   C. an antacid
   D. a mucosal protective barrier

59. The initial, **EMPIRICAL** drug of choice, based on clinical grounds, for the treatment of adult meningitis is
   A. erythromycin
   B. amphotericin B
   C. tetracycline
   D. ampicillin

60. The initial, **EMPIRICAL** drug of choice, based on clinical grounds, for the treatment of otitis media in a child less than four years of age is
   A. amoxicillin or ampicillin
   B. erythromycin plus a sulfonamide
   C. tetracycline
   D. cefaclor

61. The initial, **EMPIRICAL** drug of choice, based on clinical grounds, for the treatment of otitis media in adults is
   A. tetracycline
   B. cefaclor
   C. clindamycin
   D. ampicillin

62. The initial, **EMPIRICAL** drug of choice, based on clinical grounds, for the treatment of nongonorrheal urethritis is
    A. tetracycline
    B. ampicillin
    C. erythromycin
    D. chloramphenicol

63. The initial, **EMPIRICAL** drug of choice, based on clinical grounds, for the treatment of trichomoniasis is
    A. tetracycline
    B. penicillin
    C. metronidazole
    D. miconazole

64. The initial, **EMPIRICAL** drug of choice, based on clinical grounds, for the treatment of adults under 40 years of age with pneumonia is
    A. chloramphenicol
    B. miconazole
    C. erythromycin
    D. amphotericin B

65. The initial, **EMPIRICAL** drug of choice, based on clinical grounds, for the treatment of exudative pharyngitis is
    A. penicillin V
    B. tetracycline
    C. trimethoprim/sulfoxazole
    D. chloramphenicol

66. The initial, **EMPIRICAL** drug of choice, based on clinical grounds, for the treatment of acute sinusitis is
    A. cefaclor
    B. amoxicillin clavulanate
    C. erythromycin
    D. cefixime

67. The initial, **EMPIRICAL** drug of choice, based on clinical grounds, for the treatment of uncomplicated cystitis is
   A. penicillin G
   B. penicillin V
   C. trimethoprim/sulfoxazole
   D. erythromycin

68. The initial, **EMPIRICAL** drug of choice, based on clinical grounds, for the treatment on nonbullous impetigo is
   A. penicillin V
   B. tetracycline
   C. cefixime
   D. chloramphenicol

69. The initial, **EMPIRICAL** drug of choice, based on clinical grounds, for the treatment of Rocky Mountain spotted fever is
   A. a sulfonamide
   B. ampicillin
   C. trimethoprim/sulfoxazole
   D. doxycycline

70. The initial, **EMPIRICAL** drug of choice, based on clinical grounds, for the prophylactic treatment of a human bite is
   A. tetracycline
   B. amoxicillin clavulanate
   C. dicloxacillin
   D. cloxacillin

71. The initial, **EMPIRICAL** drug of choice, based on clinical grounds, for the prophylactic treatment of a dog bite is
   A. penicillin V
   B. erythromycin
   C. cloxacillin
   D. dicloxacillin

72. The initial, **EMPIRICAL** drug of choice, based on clinical grounds, for the treatment of Lyme disease (stage 1) is
   A. tetracycline
   B. ceftriaxone
   C. penicillin G
   D. amphotericin B

73. Which drug may be effective in the treatment of genital herpes?
   A. Amantadine
   B. 5-Fluorouracil
   C. Rimantadine
   D. Acyclovir

74. Which of the following may be effective in the treatment of human papilloma virus?
   A. Amantadine
   B. Rimantadine
   C. Podophyllin(25%)
   D. Acyclovir

75. Which of the following should **NOT** be used in pediatric patients?
   A. Penicillin
   B. Tetracycline
   C. Erythromycin
   D. Cefaclor

76. Which is **TRUE** about cephalosporins and penicillin-allergic patients?
   A. Early experiments indicated almost no cross-allergenicity
   B. The risk of reaction to cephalosporins is less than 2%
   C. There is less indication for the newer cephalosporins as an alternative than the first generation
   D. Any patient who is proven penicillin-sensitive by skin test cannot be given a cephalosporin

77. Prothrombin time can be increased in oral anticoagulant therapy by
   A. an aminoglycoside
   B. trimethoprim/sulfamethoxazole
   C. a sulfonamide
   D. quinine
   E. all of the above

78. Which of the following has/have an adverse effect on digoxin?
   A. Amoxicillin
   B. Cephalothin
   C. Doxycycline
   D. Dicloxacillin
   E. All of the above

DIRECTIONS (Questions 79–105): For each of the questions or incomplete statements below, **one or more** of the answers or completions given are correct. Select:

  A   if only **1, 2,** and **3** are correct,
  B   if only **1** and **3** are correct,
  C   if only **2** and **4** are correct,
  D   if only **4** is correct,
  E   if **all** are correct.

79. Which of the following is/are cardioselective beta-blocker(s)?
    1. Propranolol (Inderal)
    2. Nadolol (Corgard)
    3. Pindolol (Visken)
    4. Atenolol (Tenormin)

80. Which of the following is/are **TRUE** concerning beta-blockers?
    1. Increase myocardial contractility
    2. Decrease cardiac output
    3. Increase conduction velocity
    4. Decrease heart rate

81. Beta-blockers can be used to treat
    1. hypertension
    2. angina
    3. arrhythmia
    4. migraine

82. Contraindications to the use of beta-blockers include(s)
    1. congestive heart failure
    2. patients over age 65
    3. A-V node conduction disturbances
    4. concurrent diuretic use

83. Which have combined beta- and alpha-blocking activity?
    1. Metoprolol (Lopressor)
    2. Timolol (Blocadren)
    3. Nadolol (Corgard)
    4. Labetalol (Trandate)

		Directions Summarized		
A	**B**	**C**	**D**	**E**
1,2,3	1,3	2,4	4	All are
only	only	only	only	correct

84. Which of the following is/are potassium sparing diuretic(s)?
1. Hydrochlorothiazide (HydroDiuril)
2. Triamterene (Dyrenium)
3. Chlorthalidone (Hygroton)
4. Spironolactone (Aldactone)

85. The **MOST** effective diuretic category(ies) is/are the
1. potassium-sparing diuretics
2. thiazide-like diuretics
3. thiazide diuretics
4. loop diuretics

86. Thiazide diuretics are generally **NOT** recommended in the treatment of hypertension for which of the following?
1. Patients with renal insufficiency
2. Patients with high plasma levels of renin
3. Patients with hypersensitivity reactions to thiazides
4. Patients with essential hypertension

87. Which is/are **TRUE** about hypertensive treatment with vasodilators such as hydralazine and minoxidil?
1. Orthostatic hypotension is not a problem
2. Impotence is not a common side-effect
3. Decrease peripheral vascular resistance
4. Sympathetic reflexes reduce effectiveness

88. Treatment of the failing heart with digitalis increases
1. stroke volume
2. cardiac contractility
3. vagomimetic influences
4. heart rate

89. Clinical uses of digitalis include management of
    1. Type 1 second degree A-V block bradycardia
    2. congestive heart failure
    3. cardiac failure secondary to mechanical obstruction
    4. most supraventricular arrhythmias

90. Adverse reactions to digitalis
    1. occur in 20% of digitalized hospital patients
    2. are potentially lethal
    3. are greater in patients with advanced heart disease
    4. are exacerbated by hyperkalemia

91. Which of the following increase(s) digoxin half-life?
    1. Quinidine
    2. Corticosteroids
    3. Verapamil
    4. Antacids

92. The therapeutic objectives in the treatment of angina pectoris are to
    1. terminate acute attacks
    2. prevent acute attacks
    3. increase exercise capacity
    4. decrease coronary artery compliance

93. The effect of nitroglycerin in the treatment of angina involves
    1. transient dilation of coronary vessels
    2. reduction of ventricular pressure
    3. reduction in cardiac preload and afterload
    4. no change in heart rate

94. Adverse reactions to nitroglycerin include
    1. esophageal spasm
    2. postural hypotension
    3. muscle cramps
    4. vascular headaches

95. Nitroglycerin may be taken or used
    1. topically
    2. intravenously
    3. sublingually
    4. orally

		Directions Summarized		
A	**B**	**C**	**D**	**E**
1,2,3	1,3	2,4	4	All are
only	only	only	only	correct

96. Which of the following is/are calcium channel blockers?
   1. Verapamil (Calan)
   2. Nifedipine (Procardia)
   3. Diltiazem (Cardizem)
   4. Dipyridamole (Persantine)

97. Calcium channel blockers may be used to treat
   1. some cardiac arrhythmias
   2. hypertension
   3. angina
   4. low-salt induced muscle cramps

98. Which is **NOT** true of calcium channel blockers?
   1. Verapamil is very effective in the acute control of PSVT
   2. Contraindicated in angina caused by coronary vasospasm
   3. Can be effectively combined with long-acting nitrates
   4. High incidence of side-effects

99 Which of the following is/are **TRUE** of nifedipine (Procardia)?
   1. Has a vasodilator action
   2. Cannot be used for antihypertensive treatment
   3. Hypotensive effect is well sustained during therapy
   4. Efficacy is increased with concurrent beta-blocker use

100. Quinidine is contraindicated in which of the following conditions?
   1. Complete A-V block
   2. Congestive heart failure
   3. Hypotension
   4. Myasthenia gravis

101. Which of the following is/are **TRUE** about bretylium?
   1. First line antiarrhythmic
   2. Available in oral and parenteral forms
   3. Used as a long-term antiarrhythmic
   4. Used to treat life-threatening ventricular arrhythmias

102. Primary indications for the use of erythromycin include
1. *Mycoplasma pneumoniae*
2. gonorrhea
3. pediatric otitis media
4. syphilis

103. Benefits of early treatment in the initial episode of genital herpes with acyclovir (Zovirax) include
1. reduced viral shedding
2. increased healing of lesions
3. decreased duration of pain
4. decreased new lesion formation

104. Which of the following is/are **TRUE** of metronidazole (Flagyl)?
1. FDA approved for the treatment of trichomoniasis and amebiasis
2. 250 mg tid for seven days is highly effective for trichomoniasis
3. Alcohol should be avoided during treatment
4. No treatment of partners is necessary if patient is sexually inactive during treatment period

105. Drugs used in the termination of acute gout include
1. aspirin
2. indomethacin
3. acetaminophen
4. colchicine

Explanatory Answers

36. A. A fundamental concept of pharmacology is the interaction of a drug and a cell receptor that causes a change in the receptor that results in a response. (Ref. 2, p. 9)

37. B. An agonist initiates a response. (Ref. 2, p. 10)

38. A. An antagonist has no biological effect of its own, but causes a reaction by inhibiting the normal response at the receptor site. (Ref. 2, p. 10)

39. D. The measurement of drug disappearance is the biological half-life. It is an estimate of the time required to reduce the quantity of drug present in a particular body compartment. (Ref. 2, p. 39)

40. E. The principal organ systems involved in drug excretion are listed, with the kidneys being the primary organ for most drugs. (Ref. 2, p. 59)

41. E. The volume of drug distribution is the location of the drug in the body and is not a renal factor in excretion. (Ref. 2, p. 63)

42. D. Phase 1 studies are designed to establish the dose level at which signs of toxicity first appear and involve healthy males. (Ref. 2, p. 112)

43. A. Phase 2 studies are designed to evaluate efficacy and to establish optimal dose range. (Ref. 2, p. 113)

44. C. Adverse reactions are an important component of all phases. (Ref. 2, p. 113)

45. D. Phase 4 studies allow continued evaluation by controlled or uncontrolled studies, and may include groups excluded from previous studies. (Ref. 2, p. 113)

46. B. Platelet counts should also be obtained and followed. (Ref. 2, p. 373)

47. E.   Lab values vary, but generally 1.5 to 2 times normal is acceptable. (Ref. 2, p. 374)

48. D.   Salicylates increase the effect of warfarin by inhibition of clotting factors and platelet adhesiveness. The other choices decrease the anticoagulant effect. (Ref. 2, p. 377)

49. A.   Antimicrobials work in all the modes listed; but, only choice A is true for the penicillins and cephalosporins. (Ref. 2, p. 654)

50. D.   The tetracyclines are bacteriostatic, rather than bactericidal. (Ref. 2, p. 687)

51. E.   It is generally accepted that the above organisms are susceptible to the penicillins unless proven resistant. (Ref. 2, pp. 654–679)

52. B.   The cephalosporins, particularly the third generation, are considered broad spectrum. (Ref. 2, pp. 654–679)

53. C.   Erythromycin is effective against a broad spectrum of organisms. (Ref. 2, pp. 692–695)

54. D.   Cimetidine can be given orally with its major use in the treatment of gastric and duodenal ulcers and hypersecretory states such as Zollinger-Ellison syndrome. It competes for H_2 receptor sites. (Ref. 2, p. 969)

55. D.   Probenecid blocks the active reabsorption of uric acid in the proximal tubules. It is not useful during the acute phase of gout, but will decrease the incidence of attacks. (Ref. 2, pp. 596–597)

56. A.   Cromolyn sodium is effective only when used prophylactically and is not indicated in the management of acute bronchospasm. (Ref. 2, pp. 601–612)

57. E.   Salicylates should be the first line of pharmacologic treatment in the effort to reduce pain and inflammation. (Ref. 2, p. 570)

58. D.   Sucralfate has an affinity for ulcerative craters and forms a protective barrier. (Ref. 2, p. 988)

59. D.   Another primary choice is penicillin G. Alternative choices are ceftriaxone, cefotaxime, or chloramphenicol. (Ref. 3, p. 4)

60. B.   An alternative choice is cefaclor. (Ref. 3, p. 6)

61. D.   Additional primary choices include trimethoprim/sulfamethoxazole, amoxicillin clavulante, cefuroxime, or cefixime. An alternative is cefaclor. (Ref. 3, p. 6)

62. A.   The other primary choice is doxycycline. An alternative is erythromycin. (Ref. 3, p. 13)

63. C.   Metronidazole is contraindicated in pregnancy. An alternative is a 20% saline douche. (Ref. 3, p. 16)

64. C.   An alternative is doxycycline. (Ref. 3, p. 22)

65. A.   Another primary choice is penicillin G, IM. An alternative is erythromycin. (Ref. 3, p. 26)

66. B.   Other primary choices are trimethoprim/sulfisoxazole or cefuroxime. Alternatives are ampicillin or cefixime. (Ref. 3, p. 26)

67. C.   Alternatives are amoxicillin, trimethoprim, or doxycycline. (Ref. 3, p. 20)

68. A.   Alternatives are erythromycin or a first-generation cephalosporin, but not cefixime. (Ref. 3, p. 28)

69. D.   Another primary choice is tetracycline. An alternative is chloramphenicol. Sulfonamides and trimethoprim/sulfoxazole should be avoided. (Ref. 3, p. 31)

70. B.   Other primary choices include penicillin V, ampicillin, or clindamycin. Alternatives include cefoxitin or erythromycin. (Ref. 3, p. 29)

71. A.   Another primary choice is ampicillin. Alternatives include tetracycline, amoxicillin clavulanate, or ceftriaxone. (Ref. 3, p. 29)

72. A.   Alternatives include penicillin V or erythromycin. Penicillin V is the drug of choice in children and pregnant women. Ceftriaxone is used to treat in stage 2 or 3, with penicillin G as an alternative. (Ref. 3, p. 30)

73. D.   Of the choices, only acyclovir is beneficial in the treatment of herpes. (Ref. 3, p. 98)

74. C.   Other primary choices include 50% trichloroacetic acid and interferon alfa-2b. 5-Fluorouracil cream may be used in the vagina. (Ref. 3, p. 98)

75. B.   Tetracycline may cause dental abnormalities in pediatric patients. (Ref. 3, p. 98)

76. B.   Early investigations suggested significant cross-allergenicity between the penicillins and cephalosporins. The newer cephalosporins may now be an alternative in penicillin-sensitive patients. There are studies of penicillin-sensitive individuals who had no reactions to cephalosporins. (Ref. 3, p. 102)

77. E.   All the drugs listed may increase the effect of the oral anticoagulants. (Ref. 3, pp. 110–113)

78. C.   Doxycycline will increase the serum levels of digoxin. (Ref. 3, pp. 110–113)

79. D.   Atenolol (Tenormin) is cardioselective. (Ref. 2, p. 165)

80. C.   Beta-blockers decrease heart rate, myocardial contractility, cardiac output, and conduction velocity. (Ref. 2, pp. 164–166)

81. E.   Beta-blockers can be used clinically to treat hypertension, angina, arrhythmias, hyperthyroidism, glaucoma, anxiety states, and migraine headaches. (Ref. 2, pp. 167–168)

82. B.   Patients with the signs and symptoms of congestive heart failure and conduction disturbances should not be given beta-blockers. Additionally, beta-blockers should be used with caution in asthmatics and diabetics, and, if indicated, only cardioselective beta-blockers should be used. (Ref. 2, p. 168)

83. E.   Labetalol is useful for the chronic treatment of primary hypertension and its effects are primarily beta. (Ref. 2, pp. 169–171)

84. C.   The potassium sparing diuretics, generally used in combination with other diuretics, are triamterene, spironolactone, and amiloride HCl. (Ref. 2, pp. 265–268)

85. D.   The loop or high ceiling diuretics have the highest efficacy for inducing marked water and electrolyte excretion. (Ref. 2, pp. 268–269)

86. A.   Thiazides should be avoided in patients with the first three conditions. (Ref. 2, pp. 272–273)

87. E.   All points are true of vasodilators in the treatment of hypertension. (Ref. 2, pp. 276–279)

88. A.   Digitalis increases the speed and force of cardiac muscle fibers. Stroke volume (and therefore cardiac output) is increased. Blood volume, venous pressure and end-diastolic pressure are reduced. Reflexive tachycardia is abolished and heart rate is also decreased by vagomimetic influences. (Ref. 2, pp. 311–313)

89. C.   Digitalis can be used in the management of congestive heart failure, most supraventricular arrhythmias, and reducing ventricular rate in atrial flutter or fibrillation. (Ref. 2, p. 314)

90. E.   Adverse reactions to digitalis are common and potentially lethal. The role of potassium is a major component in digitalis toxicity. (Ref. 2, pp. 315–316)

91. B.   Numerous substances affect the half-life and effect of digoxin. (Ref. 2, p. 318)

92. A.   By reducing myocardial oxygen demand or by increasing oxygen supply, attacks of angina can be prevented and terminated, and patient exercise tolerance can be increased. (Ref. 2, pp. 324–325)

93. A.   The exact mechanism of nitroglycerin is unknown, but NTG causes peripheral dilation that results in reduced preload and afterload, and a decrease in ventricular pressure. The effect on coronary vessels is investigational, but dilation does occur to some degree, particularly at epicardial stenotic sites. (Ref. 2, pp. 326–327)

94. C. Common side effects of organic nitrates include vascular headache and postural hypotension. (Ref. 2, p. 328)

95. E. NTG may be delivered by the routes listed. (Ref. 2, pp. 328–329)

96. A. Dipyridamole is a nonnitrate coronary vasodilator. (Ref. 2, p. 299)

97. A. Calcium channel blockers are currently used to treat some arrhythmias, hypertension, and angina. There are indications that they may be useful in treating asthma, migraine, arterial disease, and cardiomyopathy. (Ref. 2, pp. 303–305)

98. C. Verapamil has an 80% success rate in the treatment of PSVT. The calcium channel blockers have a very low frequency of side effects that are generally minor. They are beneficial in the treatment of angina caused by vasospasm and can be used with long-acting nitrates. (Ref. 2, pp. 299–306)

99. B. The calcium channel blockers reduce peripheral resistance by vasodilation, making them useful as antihypertensives. The antihypertensive effect is well sustained during therapy and can be enhanced when combined with beta-blockers. (Ref. 2, pp. 302–305)

100. E. The negative inotropic action of quinidine may depress cardiac action as well as affect the myoneural junctions. (Ref. 2, p. 343)

101. D. Bretylium is useful in the treatment of life-threatening ventricular arrhythmias that are unresponsive to lidocaine or procainamide. It is available for parenteral use only, and use should not exceed five days. (Ref. 2, p. 365)

102. B. The relatively few primary indications for erythromycin include *M. pneumoniae,* Legionnaires' disease, and diptheria. It is a popular choice for pediatric otitis media because *H. influenzae* and *S. pneumoniae* are usually sensitive. It is a second-line choice for the treatment of syphilis and gonorrhea. (Ref. 2, p. 693)

103. E. Acyclovir is particularly effective in the treatment of initial episodes of genital herpes, and less effective in recurrent episodes. (Ref. 2, p. 719)

104. A. Sexual partners should be treated concurrently. (Ref. 2, pp. 725–726)

105. C. A variety of NSAIDs or colchicine will relieve acute episodes of gout. (Ref. 2, pp. 593–594)

3 Psychiatry

DIRECTIONS (Questions 106–140): Each of the questions or incomplete statements below is followed by four or five suggested answers or completions. Select the **one** that is best in each case.

106. A false belief firmly held, despite solid proof or evidence to the contrary, is called a(n)
  A. hallucination
  B. delusion
  C. neologism
  D. idea of reference

107. The rapid progression or "racing" of thoughts with poor logical connection is called
  A. flight of ideas
  B. tangentiality
  C. blocking
  D. clanging

108. DSM III-R is a widely used system for
  A. identifying the causes of abnormal behavior
  B. distinguishing sanity from insanity
  C. identifying treatment approaches for psychiatric disorders
  D. classifying psychiatric disorders

109. Sharon is afraid to admit to herself that she hates her sister. Instead, she wrongly believes her sister hates her. This is an example of which defense mechanism?
   A. Projection
   B. Denial
   C. Intellectualization
   D. Rejection

110. The exclusion of unacceptable unconscious impulses from consciousness is called
   A. regression
   B. displacement
   C. repression
   D. rationalization

111. Immediately after losing his job of many years, Steve feels very little, but talks a great deal about the general pros and cons of staying with one company for so long. This could well be an example of which defense mechanism?
   A. Regression
   B. Displacement
   C. Reaction formation
   D. Intellectualization

112. Rigid, unjustifiably suspicious, excessively self-important personality is
   A. narcissistic
   B. paranoid
   C. schizotypal
   D. borderline

113. A personality disorder is
   A. any psychological disorder or abnormality
   B. characterized by two or more alternating personalities
   C. the label we attach to relatively minor disorders such as situational adjustment problems
   D. characterized by deeply ingrained, inflexible, maladaptive ways of dealing with reality

114. Dyspareunia refers to
    A. spastic vaginal contractions
    B. painful intercourse
    C. a physical condition involving adhesions on the clitoris
    D. a woman who has never experienced orgasm (either from masturbation or intercourse)

115. If a man has had a history of intromission, but is presently unable to achieve an erection sufficient for intercourse, he likely is suffering from
    A. primary impotence
    B. ejaculatory inhibition
    C. situational orgasmic dysfunction
    D. secondary erectile dysfunction

116. With regard to the research by Masters and Johnson, the typical order of the sexual response cycle is
    A. excitement, plateau, resolution, orgasm
    B. arousal, orgasm, refraction, resolution
    C. excitement, plateau, orgasm, resolution
    D. excitement, plateau, refraction, orgasm

117. Sensate focus is to erectile dysfunction as the squeeze technique is to
    A. ejaculatory incompetence
    B. vaginismus
    C. erectile dysfunction
    D. premature ejaculation

118. Which of the following is NOT one of the paraphilias?
    A. Pedophilia
    B. Frigidity
    C. Transvestism
    D. Sadomasochism

119. Affective disorders are characterized primarily by disturbances in
    A. thought
    B. behavior
    C. mood
    D. communication

120. What do amnesia, fugue, and multiple personality have in common?
   A. They involve physical symptoms with no organic cause
   B. They involve a splitting off of a part of personality
   C. They are characterized by disturbances of mood
   D. They can be treated with drug therapy

121. Which of the following is **NOT** a symptom of depression?
   A. Loss of energy
   B. Feelings of worthlessness
   C. Amnesia
   D. Difficulty in thinking

122. Which of the following is characterized by persistent, irrational fear of a specific object or situation?
   A. Generalized anxiety disorder
   B. Hypochondriacal disorder
   C. Phobic disorder
   D. Posttraumatic stress disorder

123. John, an accountant, complains that he feels apprehensive and fearful most of the time, but does not know why. Without much warning, his heart will begin to pound, his hands get cold, and he will break out in a sweat. He **MOST** likely suffers from which of the following disorders?
   A. Obsessive-compulsive
   B. Phobic
   C. Somatoform
   D. Generalized anxiety

124. Disorders in which conscious awareness becomes separated from previous memories, thoughts, and feelings are called
   A. affective disorders
   B. dissociative disorders
   C. somatoform disorders
   D. schizophrenic disorders

125. Rachel feels sad and believes she will never again do the things she once enjoyed. She is apathetic, does not eat, reports being tired all the time, and spends most of the day just sitting and staring. Her symptoms would probably be diagnosed as
    A. manic-depressive disorder
    B. depersonalization disorder
    C. depression
    D. schizoid personality disorder

126. An anxiety disorder characterized by unwanted repetitive thoughts and actions is called a(n)
    A. dissociative disorder
    B. obsessive-compulsive disorder
    C. schizophrenic disorder
    D. delusional disorder

127. Bipolar disorder is to affective disorders as which of the following is to somatoform disorders?
    A. Depression
    B. Panic attack
    C. Fugue
    D. Conversion disorder

128. Mr. Walker believes that he is President of the United States and that he will soon become the "King of the Universe." Mr. Walker is likely suffering from which of the following schizophrenias?
    A. Catatonic
    B. Undifferentiated
    C. Disorganized
    D. Paranoid

129. Phobic disorder is to anxiety disorders as fugue is to which of the following disorders?
    A. Dissociative
    B. Conversion
    C. Affective
    D. Somatoform

130. The **MOST** common form of hallucination is
    A. seeing visions
    B. feeling strange bodily sensations
    C. smelling unusual odors
    D. hearing voices

131. When an individual experiences genuine physical symptoms such as blindness or paralysis, but the situation reveals no physiological basis, he/she is likely suffering from a
    A. somatoform disorder
    B. dissociative disorder
    C. generalized anxiety disorder
    D. bipolar disorder

132. Which of the following is **NOT** included as a "vegetative" symptom of depression?
    A. Sleep disturbance
    B. Decreased libido
    C. Depressed mood
    D. Psychomotor retardation

133. Which of the following is **NOT** a characteristic of a manic disorder?
    A. Distractibility
    B. Delusions and hallucinations
    C. Decreased self-esteem
    D. Decreased need for sleep

134. Which of the following is **NOT** a characteristic of a schizoid personality disorder?
    A. Socially withdrawn and introverted
    B. No eccentricities of speech, behavior, or thought
    C. Hypersensitive to praise or criticism or to the feelings of others
    D. Diminished libido

135. A person who consistently exhibits little remorse for wrongdoing, even toward friends and family members, would **MOST** likely be diagnosed as having a(n)
    A. antisocial personality disorder
    B. schizotypal personality disorder
    C. schizophrenia
    D. dissociative disorder

136. Systematic desensitization is a behavioral treatment technique widely used in modern psychiatry for which one of the following conditions?
    A. Dissociative disorders
    B. Phobic disorders
    C. Conversion disorders
    D. Generalized anxiety disorders

137. Antidepressant medication is most helpful for (ie, most likely to respond to) all of the following symptoms **EXCEPT**
    A. sleep disturbance
    B. hopelessness
    C. psychomotor retardation/agitation
    D. decreased libido

138. Antipsychotic medication is most helpful for (ie, most likely to respond to) all of the following symptoms **EXCEPT**
    A. combativeness
    B. hallucinations
    C. sleeplessness
    D. poor judgment

139. Use of antipsychotic medication can cause all of the following **EXCEPT**
    A. EKG changes
    B. akathisia
    C. increased seizure threshold
    D. decreased blood pressure

140. All of the following are true regarding antidepressant medications
EXCEPT
 A. prescribing these drugs can help patients with sleep
 disturbances
 B. these medications tend to elevate the patient's mood within
 an average of 2 to 4 hours
 C. anticholinergic side-effects are common
 D. ingesting large doses of these medications can prove to be
 lethal

Explanatory Answers

106. B. Delusions are classic examples of disturbances of thought content and are often present with or suggestive of psychotic illness. (Ref. 4, p. 65)

107. A. Commonly seen in manic patients, flight of ideas represents a disturbance of thought process. Speech is fragmented and associations are determined by chance or temporal factors. (Ref. 4, p. 64)

108. D. Developed by the American Psychiatric Association, DSM III-R is the accepted means of classifying psychiatric disorders and is done on the basis of specific patterns of abnormal behavior. (Ref. 4, p. 50)

109. A. Projection is one of the basic defense mechanisms identified by Freud, whereby motives and feelings unacceptable to the self are unconsciously attributed to others instead. (Ref. 4, p. 31)

110. C. According to Freud, repression is perhaps the most basic and fundamental mechanism of defense. It involves forcing thoughts, memories, and feelings into the unconscious and keeping them out of awareness. (Ref. 4, p. 30)

111. D. Another psychological defense mechanism, intellectualization is a subtle form of denial whereby we detach ourselves from our problems by analyzing them to an extreme, almost as if they concerned other people and did not bother us emotionally. (Ref. 4, p. 32)

112. B. Paranoia refers to a pervasive and unwarranted suspiciousness and mistrust of others. Individuals with this sort of personality constantly remain on guard towards others, are overconcerned with power and rank, and tend to feel that their view of the world is the only correct one. (Ref. 4, p. 142)

113. D. Personality disorders are longstanding, maladaptive ways of relating to the world. Individuals with such problems tend to experience difficulties in social and vocational areas, and commonly feel the problems do not lie within themselves, but in the environment. (Ref. 4, p. 138)

114. B. Dyspareunia refers to pain in the genital area during intercourse. It is more common in women; there can be both physical and psychological causes for this problem. (Ref. 4, p. 229)

115. D. One of the most common sexual problems for men, erectile dysfunction or impotence is an inability to achieve and maintain an erection sufficient for intercourse. Causes for this difficulty can be organic or psychological. Care is needed in discussing sexual difficulties (with men and women) due to feelings of sensitivity and low self-esteem. (Ref. 4, p. 229)

116. C. Detailed sexological research has identified this four-phase cycle, which represents a continuum of physiological arousal during sexual stimulation. (Ref. 4, p. 222)

117. D. Sensate focus represents a treatment technique commonly used for problems of erectile dysfunction. Similarly, the squeeze technique (and also the "stop-and-go" techniques) are treatment strategies for dealing with premature ejaculation. (Ref. 4, p. 234)

118. B. "Frigidity" or general sexual dysfunction (sometimes involving problems of aversion or arousal) refers to an inability in women to derive erotic pleasure from sexual stimulation. It is classified as a psychosexual dysfunction. The other three disorders are classified as paraphilias or psychosexual deviation disorders. (Ref. 4, pp. 227, 237)

119. C. By definition, "affect" refers to mood. This group of disorders is primarily characterized by disturbances in mood, ranging from deep depression to uncontrolled elation and mania. (Ref. 4, p. 101)

120. B. These psychiatric problems are classified as dissociative disorders and involve a dissociation, separation, or splitting off of a part of personality. They may take the form of memory loss, change in identity, or presence of several distinct personality patterns. (Ref. 4, p. 191)

121. C. Amnesia or memory loss is more characteristic of organic or dissociative disorders. The symptoms of depression usually involve mood, behavior, and cognition (eg, sense of guilt, worthlessness, difficulty concentrating). (Ref. 4, p. 104)

122. C. A phobia is a persistent and irrational fear of a specific object, activity, or situation that results in a compelling desire to avoid what is feared. (Ref. 4, p. 182)

123. D. Generalized anxiety disorders are usually nonspecific (ie, do not involve a specific object or situation) and are characterized by pervasive feelings of apprehensiveness and vigilance, and include symptoms of motor tension and autonomic hyperactivity. (Ref. 4, p. 181)

124. B. These disorders involve a dissociation or splitting off of personality and are often due to experiencing a major psychological trauma. The resulting problems can include difficulties in memory, identity, or the presence of multiple personalities. (Ref. 4, p. 191)

125. C. Classic signs of depression can include depressed mood, problems with appetite-sleep-energy, loss of interest in usual activities (anhedonia), and feelings of hopelessness and worthlessness. (Ref. 4, p. 104)

126. B. Obsessions are persistent unwanted thoughts or images that force themselves into one's mind. Compulsions are repetitive urges to perform certain acts that are contrary to one's wishes or standards. In some individuals, both patterns can take on a strong compulsive quality that can eventually interfere with everyday living and generate much anxiety. (Ref. 4, p. 170)

127. D. A bipolar disorder (ie, manic depression) involves the experiencing of severe mood swings or problems in affect. A conversion disorder is a type of somatoform disorder whereby physical symptoms of serious body dysfunction occur, but in the absence of any genuine physical evidence or organic cause (eg, paralysis, blindness). (Ref. 4, p. 187)

128. D. Schizophrenia is characterized by significant disturbances in thought, behavior, speech, and mood. The paranoid type involves the presence of grandiose, jealous, or persecutory delusions, or hallucinations with persecutory or grandiose content. (Ref. 4, p. 88)

129. A. Phobias are classified under anxiety disorders due to the primary characteristic of experiencing high levels of anxiety. Fugue (amnesia combined with physical flight and including the assumption of a new identity) is classified under dissociative disorders because of the characteristic of splitting off or dissociating part of one's personality. (Ref. 4, pp. 182, 191)

130. D. Hallucinations are perceptions believed to be real, despite evidence to the contrary (ie, an individual perceives something that does not exist). They can be experienced through any of the senses, but the most common are auditory hallucinations (usually of a persecutory or condemning nature). (Ref. 4, p. 68)

131. A. Somatoform disorders are psychiatric disorders that assume the form of somatic illness. All are characterized by physical symptoms that cannot be accounted for by any demonstrable physical evidence (eg, somatization disorder, conversion disorder, psychogenic pain disorder, hypochondriasis). (Ref. 4, pp. 187–191)

132. C. "Vegetative" symptoms refer to specific physical problems that often accompany a depression. These include: sleep disturbance, appetite disturbance, loss of energy, decreased libido, and psychomotor retardation/agitation. Depressed mood per se would be an "affective" symptom of a depression. (Ref. 4, p. 104)

133. C. Mania refers to a type of affective disturbance characterized by euphoria, hyperactivity, pressured speech, flight of ideas, *inflated* self-esteem, decreased need for sleep, lability of mood, distractibility, and delusions/hallucinations. (Ref. 4, p. 123)

134. C. The schizoid personality is characterized as socially withdrawn, introverted, eccentric, and uncomfortable with most forms of contact with other people. Schizoid individuals resemble schizophrenics in their odd and withdrawn manner, but do not exhibit the associated problems in disordered thinking. Commonly, they demonstrate indifference to praise or criticism or to the feelings of others. (Ref. 4, p. 145)

135. A. The antisocial personality disorder is characterized by a longstanding pattern of behavior in which the the rights of others are repeatedly violated. There is often much evidence of irritability and aggression, poor impulse control, disregard for the truth, and problems sustaining interpersonal-vocational-intimate relationships. (Ref. 4, p. 156)

136. B. Systematic desensitization is a behavior modification technique commonly used for problems that involve anxiety specific to particular situations (eg, phobias, sexual dysfunctions). It is less useful for more diffuse anxiety. The technique involves learning progressive relaxation and then applying it to a sequenced hierarchy of progressively anxiety-provoking scenes. (Ref. 4, p. 332)

137. B. The depressive symptoms most likely to be alleviated by antidepressant medication are the "vegetative" or physical signs (problems with sleep, appetite, libido, energy, movement). Less likely to respond are the subjective or psychological signs (difficulties with demoralization, self-esteem, and feelings of helplessness/hopelessness). (Ref. 4, p. 367)

138. D. The psychotic symptoms most likely to respond to neuroleptic medication are combativeness, hyperactivity, tension, hostility, hallucinations, sleeplessness, poor hygiene and self-care, acute delusions and social isolation. (Basically they improve alertness, energy, and physical awareness.) Less likely to respond to such medication are problems involving poor judgment, impaired memory, disorientation, and chronic delusions. (Ref. 4, p. 354)

139. C. Some of the notable side-effects/risks of neuroleptic medication can include sedation, _lowered_ seizure threshold, anticholinergic responses, EKG changes, postural hypotension, and extrapyramidal reactions (tic and movement disorders). (Ref. 4, p. 357)

140. B. Generally, antidepressant medication can take an average of 7 to 10 days before the patient notices significant changes in his/her symptoms. Therefore, it may be necessary to use other medications in the interim to deal with specific symptoms. (Ref. 4, pp. 366–377)

4 Geriatrics

DIRECTIONS (Questions 141–154): Each of the questions or incomplete statements below is followed by four or five suggested answers or completions. Select the **one** that is best in each case.

141. All of the following are true of presbycusis **EXCEPT**
    A. sensorineural loss
    B. loss may be compounded by cerumen impaction
    C. involves mostly low-frequency sounds
    D. mostly irreversible loss (disregarding hearing aid)

142. Senile dementia of the Alzheimer's type is a(n)
    A. multi-infarct dementia
    B. depressive pseudodementia
    C. primary degenerative dementia
    D. reversible dementia

143. Persons aged 65 and older represent approximately what percentage of patients seen in primary care practice in the United States?
    A. 10%
    B. 30%
    C. 50%
    D 75%

144. The **MOST** common cause of anemia in the elderly is
    A. anemia of chronic disease
    B. iron deficiency anemia
    C. folate deficiency anemia
    D. pernicious anemia

145. As much as 30% of the elderly population are believed to have a specific sleep disorder. The **MOST** common of these specific disorders is
    A. depression
    B. alcoholism
    C. obstructive sleep apnea
    D. drug-induced

146. In many cases, depression in the elderly patient may present with primarily physical symptoms. This is termed
    A. complex depression
    B. major depression syndrome
    C. minor depression complex
    D. masked depression

147. **MOST** dependent elderly persons in the United States are cared for by
    A. hospitals
    B. nursing homes
    C. family
    D. friends

148. Which of the following types of hip fracture in elderly patients is associated with a higher incidence of nonunion and necrosis of the femoral head?
    A. Subtrochanteric
    B. Intertrochanteric
    C. Subcapital
    D. None of the above

149. Among the numerous antiinflammatory agents useful in the treatment of musculoskeletal disorders in the elderly, the **LEAST** expensive (in terms of cost per 100 tablets) is
A. ibuprofen
B. indomethacin
C. aspirin
D. piroxicam

150. Age-related (postmenopausal) osteoporosis is associated with all of the following **EXCEPT**
A. decreased parathyroid function
B. increased incidence of vertebral fractures
C. mainly cortical bone loss
D. decreased calcium absorption

151. Cardiac auscultation of an 80-year-old man reveals a crescendo–decrescendo systolic murmur ending before the second heart sound, heard best along the lower left sternal border and apex. The murmur probably is associated with
A. mitral stenosis
B. aortic regurgitation
C. aortic stenosis
D. pulmonic regurgitation

152. An elderly patient with hypochromic anemia has low serum iron, low total iron-binding capacity, and a high ferritin level. This patient's anemia is probably which of the following?
A. Iron-deficiency anemia
B. Anemia of chronic disease
C. Sideroblastic anemia
D. Pernicious anemia

153. All of the following preventive strategies are recommended for the elderly (over age 65) **EXCEPT**
A. influenza vaccine yearly
B. cessation of smoking
C. tetanus prophylaxis every ten years
D. pneumococcal vaccine yearly

154. All of the following are true of Medicare benefits for the elderly **EXCEPT**
   A. Medicare part A is hospital insurance
   B. Medicare part B is medical insurance
   C. parts A and B involve deductibles
   D. benefits are automatic upon reaching age 65

DIRECTIONS (Questions 155–160): For each of the questions or incomplete statements below, **one or more** of the answers or completions given are correct. Select:
   A   if only **1, 2,** and **3** are correct,
   B   if only **1** and **3** are correct,
   C   if only **2** and **4** are correct,
   D   if only **4** is correct,
   E   if **all** are correct.

---

155. When performing a functional assessment of the elderly patient, the activity(s) of daily living (ADL) that should be addressed is/are
   1. dressing
   2. transfer
   3. feeding
   4. reading

156. Common detrimental changes associated with aging affect
   1. cardiac output
   2. creatinine clearance
   3. visual acuity
   4. B and T cell activity

157. Basic type(s) of persistent geriatric urinary incontinence include
   1. stress
   2. urge
   3. functional
   4. overflow

	A	B	C	D	E
Directions Summarized					
	1,2,3	1,3	2,4	4	All are
	only	only	only	only	correct

158. Common cause(s) of blindness in the elderly include(s)
1. macular degeneration
2. glaucoma
3. diabetic retinopathy
4. cataracts

159. Aging changes can be expected to affect which of the following laboratory parameters?
1. Hemoglobin and hematocrit
2. Blood urea nitrogen
3. Blood calcium
4. Blood glucose tolerance

160. Criteria for the clinical diagnosis of "probable" Alzheimer's disease include
1. deficits in two or more areas of cognition
2. no disturbance of consciousness
3. progressive worsening of memory and other cognitive functions
4. sudden, apoplectic onset

DIRECTIONS (Questions 161–165): Each group of lettered headings below is followed by a list of numbered words or phrases. For each numbered word or phrase, select:

    A   if the item is associated with **A only,**
    B   if the item is associated with **B only,**
    C   if the item is associated with **both A and B,**
    D   if the item is associated with **neither A nor B.**

    A. Delirium
    B. Dementia
    C. Both
    D. Neither

161. Attention and alertness usually normal

162. Orientation often impaired

163. Visual hallucinations relatively common

164. Onset usually insidious, rather than acute

165. Little or no memory impairment

Explanatory Answers

141. C. Presbycusis involves primarily high-frequency impairment. Frequency discrimination often becomes a problem for the elderly in relation to understanding speech, largely because consonant sounds are of higher frequency and shorter duration. (Ref. 5, pp. 309–319)

142. C. Alzheimer's dementia is a primary degenerative disorder involving alterations in the number, structure, and function of neurons in certain areas of the cerebral cortex. (Ref. 5, pp. 90–99)

143. B. Persons aged 65 and over represent 11% of the population, but represent over a third of those patients seen by primary care practitioners. (Ref. 5, pp. 19–21)

144. B. Although iron-deficiency anemia is the most common anemia seen in the elderly patient, the anemia of chronic disease may display many similarities with iron deficiency. Anemia of chronic disease is frequently associated with chronic inflammatory diseases or neoplasia. Poor dietary intake may contribute to iron deficiency in the elderly. However, even in the presence of poor nutrition, evaluation for GI bleeding should be done. Folate and B_{12} deficiency, while an important cause of anemia in the elderly, occur less often than iron-deficiency. (Ref. 5, pp. 281–285)

145. C. Obstructive sleep apnea is the most often encountered specific sleep disorder, which results not only in complaints of insomnia, but also in nighttime hypoxia with associated risks for cardiac arrhythmias, and myocardial and cerebral infarction. (Ref. 5, pp. 118–119)

146. D. Masked depression is especially common in the elderly, and may present with generalized symptoms (eg, fatigue, anorexia, weight loss) or specific complaints (eg, back pain, palpitations, abdominal pain). When elderly persons find it difficult to express directly feelings of sadness, guilt, or anger, they may somatosize these emotions and complain of physical symptoms. (Ref. 5, pp. 115–120)

147. C. Over 70% of persons aged 65 and older have surviving children, the vast majority of whom do not abandon their parents when their parents are in need of care. (Ref. 5, pp. 30–36)

148. C. Subcapital fractures (which are inside the joint capsule) disrupt the blood supply to the proximal femoral head, thus resulting in a higher probability of necrosis and nonunion. Replacement of the femoral head is often warranted in these cases. (Ref. 5, pp. 230–232)

149. C. Aspirin still remains, by far, the least expensive antiinflammatory drug. Indomethacin and ibuprofen, although much less expensive than most other NSAIDs, are 3 to 4 times more expensive than aspirin. (Ref. 5, pp. 223–225)

150. C. Postmenopausal osteoporosis usually results in trabecular bone loss, not cortical. (Ref. 5, pp. 225–229)

151. C. Aortic valve calcification is common among the elderly. In most cases, it is of no clinical significance except as a source of aortic systolic murmur. (Ref. 5, pp. 262–264)

152. B. The anemia of chronic disease may display many similarities with iron deficiency. The finding of hypochromia and low serum iron may lead to confusion with iron deficiency. Generally, a combination of low TIBC and elevated ferritin confirms the presence of anemia of chronic disease. Treatment is addressed to the underlying chronic illness. (Ref. 5, pp. 282–284)

153. D. Current evidence supports the administration of pneumococcal vaccine one time only. (Refs. 5, Ch. 15; 6, pp. 363–367)

154. D. Medicare is provided to all persons eligible for social security and others with chronic disabilities, such as end-stage renal disease. Others must pay a monthly premium if they elect to enroll in the Medicare program; coverage is not automatic for all who reach the age of 65. (Ref. 5, pp. 401–406)

155. A. The ADL assessment considers only the lower bound of functioning (eg, toiletting, bathing, feeding). Slightly more complex tasks (eg, reading, cooking, shopping) are assessed as instrumental activities of daily living (IADL). Both ADL and IADL should be evaluated in the patient's functional assessment. (Ref. 5, pp. 66–67)

156. A. Decreases in cardiac output, creatinine clearance, and visual acuity are common, but immune system deficits associated with aging occur only with T-cell, not B-cell activity. (Ref. 5, pp. 7–8)

157. E. Stress, urge, and overflow incontinence result from one or a combination of two basic lower GU tract problems: failure to store urine and/or failure to empty the bladder. Functional incontinence is seen in severe dementia and other neuropsychological disorders in which the patient is unable or unwilling to toilet. (Ref. 5, pp. 147–153)

158. E. All of the above are common visual problems in the aged which may result in blindness. Screening for these disorders should include testing visual acuity, performing an ophthalmoscopic evaluation, and checking intraocular pressure. (Ref. 5, pp. 301–308)

159. D. Normal aging changes do not affect most laboratory parameters. However, in the elderly population, 50% have glucose intolerance with normal fasting blood sugar levels. As with younger patients, abnormal lab findings in the elderly should prompt further evaluation. (Ref. 5, pp. 62, 271–274)

160. A. Sudden, apoplectic onset is not a typical feature of Alzheimer's disease. This presentation should trigger a search for systemic disorders or other brain diseases that could account for the progressive deficits in memory and cognition. (Ref. 5, p. 93)

161. B. In cases of delirium, onset is usually acute, often at night,
162. C. marked by illusions and hallucinations, abnormally high or low
163. A. states of alertness, immediate and recent memory impairment,
164. B. and varied levels of disorientation and confusion. Confusion
165. D. may also be a manifestation of dementia, particularly when associated with slowly progressive impairment of cognitive function, but not disordered alertness. (Ref. 5, pp. 84–91)

5 Substance Abuse

DIRECTIONS (Questions 166–176): Each group of lettered headings below is followed by a list of numbered words or phrases. For each numbered word or phrase, select:
A   if the item is associated with **A only,**
B   if the item is associated with **B only,**
C   if the item is associated with **both A and B,**
D   if the item is associated with **neither A nor B.**

Questions 166–169:
   A. Barbiturates
   B. Opiates
   C. Both
   D. Neither

166. As tolerance develops, the margin between lethal dose and intoxicating dose grows smaller

167. Withdrawal is highly associated with seizures and potential death

168. There is no useful test for determining the extent of dependency

169. Withdrawal symptoms mimic "flu" syndrome

Questions 170–172:
- **A.** Cocaine
- **B.** Hallucinogens
- **C.** Both
- **D.** Neither

170. Abuse can lead to psychoses

171. There is no evidence of a withdrawal syndrome

172. Intoxication causes constricted pupils and reduced body temperature

Questions 173–176:
- **A.** Wernicke's disease
- **B.** Korsakoff's disease
- **C.** Both
- **D.** Neither

173. Characterized by mental disturbance, eye movement paralysis, and ataxia

174. Most patients recover completely

175. Characterized by a defect in retention memory and learning

176. Requires immediate administration of thiamine

DIRECTIONS (Questions 177–181): The group of questions below consists of lettered headings followed by a list of numbered words, phrases, or statements. For each numbered word, phrase, or statement, select the **one** lettered heading that is most closely associated with it. Each lettered heading may be selected once, more than once, or not at all.

    A. Heroin
    B. Marijuana
    C. PCP
    D. Naloxone
    E. Cocaine

177. Preferred treatment for opiate overdose

178. One of the oldest and most widely used mind-altering drugs in the world

179. Produces detachment, disorientation, distortion of body image, loss of proprioception, and acute psychotic reactions

180. Used as a topical anesthetic in eye surgery

181. Clonidine is sometimes used to ameliorate withdrawal

DIRECTIONS (Questions 182–185): Each of the questions or incomplete statements below is followed by four or five suggested answers or completions. Select the **one** that is best in each case.

---

182. All of the following statements regarding marijuana are true **EXCEPT**
    A. almost 60% of Americans have tried marijuana at least once
    B. when marijuana is smoked, over 2,000 identifiable metabolites with unknown consequences are produced
    C. the most clearly established acute effects of marijuana are on mental functions and behavior
    D. prolonged use of marijuana causes permanent changes in the nervous system and permanently impairs brain function and behavior
    E. chronic marijuana users often outgrow their habits

183. A factor that predicted persistent heroin dependence in Vietnam veterans was
    A. amount of heroin used
    B. abuse restricted to heroin exclusively
    C. social class of abuser
    D. ethnicity of abuser
    E. lack of high school graduation

184. Leading causes of death for the alcoholic include all of the following **EXCEPT**
    A. heart disease
    B. cancer
    C. accidents
    D. pancreatitis
    E. suicide

185. U.S. states where IV drug abuse heterosexual AIDS cases exceed cases in non-IV drug abuse homosexual men include
    A. Connecticut, New Jersey, New York
    B. Connecticut, New York, Florida
    C. New York, New Jersey, Florida
    D. Missouri, New York, New Jersey
    E. Texas, New York, Florida

DIRECTIONS (Questions 186–190): For each of the questions or incomplete statements below, **one or more** of the answers or completions given are correct. Select:

    A   if only **1, 2,** and **3** are correct,
    B   if only **1** and **3** are correct,
    C   if only **2** and **4** are correct,
    D   if only **4** is correct,
    E   if **all** are correct.

186. A child suffering from fetal alcohol syndrome might exhibit which of the following defects?
1. Cardiac septal defects
2. Microcephaly
3. Poorly formed concha
4. Mental retardation

187. Which of the following statements regarding the effects of fetal exposure to cocaine is/are **TRUE**?
1. Cocaine-exposed babies have a higher rate of sudden infant death syndrome (SIDS) than narcotic-exposed babies
2. Interuterine exposure to cocaine leads to low neonatal birth weight
3. Behavioral effects, as well as physical effects, are seen in cocaine babies
4. The incidence of abruptio placenta decreases significantly in women who stop using cocaine early in pregnancy

188. Intravenous drug use associated AIDS cases are defined as cases involving
1. intravenous drug users
2. sex partners of intravenous drug users
3. children of intravenous drug users
4. children of sex partners of intravenous drug users

Directions Summarized				
A	**B**	**C**	**D**	**E**
1,2,3	1,3	2,4	4	All are
only	only	only	only	correct

189. The rate of IV drug abuse associated AIDS cases in the U.S. is highest in which of the following groups?
    1. Whites
    2. Hispanics
    3. Asian/Pacific islanders
    4. Blacks

190. Which of the following statements regarding physical dependence, or addiction, is/are **TRUE**?
    1. Its signs and symptoms are characteristic for a particular pharmacologic class of drugs
    2. It results in a withdrawal or abstinence syndrome
    3. Drug-seeking behavior is pronounced
    4. It can be described as a strong compulsion to continue or resume use of the substance

Explanatory Answers

166. A. Tolerance develops with opiates, sedative-hypnotics, stimulants, and hallucinogens. It is marked in the opiates, barbiturates, and alcohol. A concomitant increase in the lethal dose occurs as opiate tolerance occurs, but this is not true for the barbiturates. As a result, the risk for fatal overdose is particularly high in barbiturate addiction. (Ref. 7, p. 2)

167. A. A withdrawal reaction from any of the sedative-hypnotics or anxiolytic drugs may be life-threatening. Seizures occur in approximately 80% of nonmedicated patients withdrawing from short-acting barbiturates. If convulsions or seizures occur in opiate withdrawal, an undiagnosed sedative withdrawal and/or underlying medical condition such as epilepsy is indicated. (Ref. 7, p. 3)

168. B. Opiate addiction can only be diagnosed definitely upon clinical signs of withdrawal. The pentobarbital tolerance test is a reliable method, however, of determining an individual's dependency upon any of the sedative-hypnotics. (Ref. 7, p. 2)

169. B. Signs and symptoms of opiate withdrawal include rhinitis, lassitude, gastrointestinal discomfort, including vomiting and diarrhea, and muscle aches. (Ref. 9, p. 545)

170. C. Cocaine abusers may become depressed, paranoid, hyperactive, impulsive, psychotic, or suicidal. PCP and other hallucinogens can produce psychoses which require weeks to months of hospital care. (Ref. 7, pp. 5–6)

171. B. Withdrawal from cocaine includes severe depression, irritability, and anxiety. To date, withdrawal symptoms have not been noted with hallucinogens. (Ref. 7, p. 5)

172. D. Opiate and sedative-hypnotic intoxication causes constricted pupils and reduced body temperature. Cocaine causes dilated pupils and hyperthermia. The effects of hallucinogens are variable. (Ref. 7, pp. 1–6)

173. A. The ocular abnormality in Wernicke's disease is usually a sixth nerve paralysis, accompanied by horizontal diplopia, strabismus, and nystagmus. Stance and gait are affected, and about 90% of patients suffer a derangement of mental function. (Ref. 8, p. 2045)

174. D.   Most patients with either disease do not show complete recovery in one or more symptoms of the disease. (Ref. 8, p. 2046)

175. B.   Korsakoff's psychosis is the psychic component of Wernicke's disease, and is determined by the presence of amnesic symptoms. (Ref. 8, p. 2046)

176. C.   Wernicke's disease and Korsakoff's psychosis are not separate entities, but successive stages of a single disease process. Most, if not all, of the symptoms of both are due to thiamine deficiency. (Ref. 8, p. 2047)

177. D.   The opiate antagonist naloxone is the preferred treatment for OD. Initial dose is 0.4 mg IM or IV, repeated in 3 to 10 minutes if no response occurs. (Ref. 8, p. 2152)

178. B.   Cannabanoid use has been recorded for thousands of years by the eastern cultures of India and China, by the ancient Greeks, and by the Arabic nations. Approximately 200 to 300 million people use the drug in some form—30 to 40 million in the United States alone. (Ref. 9, p. 391)

179. C.   Opiates produce a "rush" followed by euphoria, tranquility, and sleepiness. Cocaine produces a "rush" described as orgasmic, followed by euphoria and a feeling of mental alertness. Inhalants produce euphoria and a "drunk" feeling, followed by disorientation, possible hallucinations, and the slow passage of time. (Ref. 9, pp. 384–393)

180. E.   In the late 1800s, Sigmund Freud fostered the use of cocaine as a stimulant and general panacea. His colleague, Karl Kolher, is believed to be the first to use it to anesthetize an eye in surgery. (Ref. 9, p. 386)

181. A.   Clonidine is thought to reduce the nervous system hyperactivity associated with narcotic withdrawal. (Ref. 2, p. 546)

182. D.   Regular heavy use of marijuana can lead to behavioral dysfunction and mental disorders, but there is no conclusive evidence to determine whether the drug is a cause or a result of these mental conditions. (Ref. 7, p. 6)

183. E. Of the 40% of enlisted men who abused heroin during the Vietnam War, only 5% continued usage on their return to the United States. Factors associated with such continued use included failure to graduate from high school, polydrug abuse, and criminal record associations that support the hypothesis that personality disorders predispose individuals to drug addiction. (Ref. 7, p. 1)

184. D. Alcoholics commonly develop acute or chronic pancreatitis, as well as other gastrointestinal problems. Most cases, with the exception of esophageal varices and atrophy of gastric cells, are reversible. (Ref. 8, p. 2148)

185. A. In 1988, 54.5% of IV drug abuse associated cases were reported from the Northeast which represents only 19.7% of the United States population. (Ref. 10, pp. 166–167)

186. E. Features of United States fetal alcohol syndrome are microcephaly, prenatal and postnatal growth deficiency, short palpebral fissures, cardiac defects, anomalies of the external genitalia and inner ear, and mental retardation. (Ref. 2, p. 539)

187. A. Cocaine abuse during pregnancy is associated with low birth weight, congenital abnormalities, and behavioral abnormalities. In one study, 15% of cocaine babies died of SIDS, whereas narcotic-exposed infants had a 4% rate of SIDS. Women discontinuing usage during the first trimester saw no decrease in the incidence of abruptio placenta. (Ref. 11, p. 291ff)

188. E. The 9,752 AIDS cases in intravenous drug users in 1988 included 5,789 male heterosexual IV drug abusers, 1,742 female heterosexual IV drug abusers, 2,055 male homosexual/bisexual IV drug abusers, 847 men and women with heterosexual IV drug abuse sex partners, and 319 children born to IV drug abusers or sex partners of IV drug abusers. (Ref. 10, p. 165)

189. D. In 1988, 18.4% of intravenous drug use associated AIDS cases occurred in blacks, 14.1% in hispanics, and 1.6% in whites. (Ref. 10, p. 166)

190. A. A strong compulsion to use a drug is the definition of psychological dependence. (Ref. 2, p. 542)

6 AIDS and Oncology

191. Which of the following describe(s) the presentation of Kaposi's sarcoma in the AIDS patient?
   1. Appear as pink, purple, and nonpigmented nodular skin lesions
   2. Are found commonly on the extremities
   3. May be associated with signs of lymphatic obstruction
   4. Skin lesions are initially painful

192. Which of the following opportunistic diseases is/are diagnostic of AIDS?
   1. Candidiasis of the esophagus, trachea, bronchi, or lungs
   2. Kaposis's sarcoma in a patient less than 60 years of age
   3. *Pneumocystis carinii* pneumonia
   4. Pulmonary *Mycobacterium tuberculosis*

193. The defects commonly seen in the immune system when associated with the HIV-1 infection are
1. abnormal B cell function
2. increased chemotaxis
3. decreased parasite killing
4. increased response to soluble antigen

194. A 23-year-old Latin American male presents in your office complaining of shortness of breath, dry hacking cough, and a temperature of 40 °C. On further questioning, the patient gives a history of hemophilia and a positive HIV ELISA test one year ago. Which of the following should be included in your differential diagnosis?
1. Cytomegalovirus (CMV) pneumonitis
2. Viral pneumonia
3. *P. carinii* pneumonia
4. Pulmonary tuberculosis

195. In an HIV-1 positive patient, a chest x-ray which shows diffuse bilateral interstitial infiltrates supports which of the following diagnoses?
1. Pulmonary tuberculosis
2. Cytomegalovirus pneumonitis
3. *Streptococcus pneumoniae* pneumonia
4. *P. carinii* pneumonia

196. Kaposi's sarcoma commonly presents in the
1. central nervous system
2. skin
3. bone
4. viscera

197. Goals of the clinical evaluation of patients infected with HIV-1 include
1. rapid identification of all treatable infectious diseases
2. isolation of all patients who are HIV-1 positive
3. evaluation of the immune system
4. avoidance of high-risk groups

		Directions Summarized		
A	**B**	**C**	**D**	**E**
1,2,3	1,3	2,4	4	All are
only	only	only	only	correct

198. In 1991, zidovudine (Retrovir or AZT) is initiated in the HIV$^+$ patient when which of the following conditions are present?
    1. T4 (CD4) count less than 200 mm^3
    2. Diagnosis with *P. carinii* pneumonia
    3. Diagnosis with CNS toxoplasmosis and T4 (CD4) count less than 200 mm^3
    4. T4 (CD4) count less than 500 mm^3

199. When conducting a history on an individual infected with HIV-1, which of the following would be beneficial to know?
    1. Comprehensive review of systems
    2. History of sexually transmitted diseases
    3. HIV-1 risk factors
    4. Immunizations as a child

200. Causes of pulmonary pathology in the AIDS patient includes
    1. Atypical mycobacteriosis
    2. Cryptococcosis
    3. *P. carinii*
    4. Coccidioidomycosis

201. A 39-year-old white male who is HIV$^+$ and has a CD4 count less than 200 mm^3 presents with a two-day history of increased dizziness on ambulation, left-sided weakness, severe frontal headaches, and fevers. Which of the following should be included in the differential diagnosis?
    1. Brainstem lymphoma
    2. Cryptococcal meningitis
    3. *Toxoplasma* encephalitis
    4. AIDS dementia complex

202. Laboratory test(s) which may be helpful to determine the progression of the HIV infection include(s)
   1. beta-2-microglobulin
   2. HIV-ELISA
   3. absolute T4 count
   4. serology for CMV

203. Drugs useful in the treatment of CNS *Toxoplasma* include
   1. amphotericin B
   2. sulfadiazine
   3. 5-flucytosine
   4. pyrimethamine

204. Treatment options for oral candidiasis include
   1. nystatin
   2. clotrimazole
   3. ketoconazole
   4. fluconazole

205. Common side-effects of zidovudine include
   1. anemia
   2. macrocytosis
   3. nausea
   4. headaches

206. Treatment options for *P. carinii* pneumonia include
   1. trimethoprim/sulfamethoxazole
   2. trimethoprim-dapsone
   3. pentamidine isethionate
   4. penicillin

207. The initial workup of a symptomatic HIV⁺ individual includes
   1. serology for CMV, EBV, HSV, and *Toxoplasma*
   2. MRI of the brain
   3. absolute T4 count
   4. p24 antigen

Directions Summarized				
A	**B**	**C**	**D**	**E**
1,2,3	1,3	2,4	4	All are
only	only	only	only	correct

208. Acute cryptococcal meningitis may be treated by prescribing
    1. amphotericin B
    2. cleocin
    3. fluconazole
    4. ketoconazole

209. The differential diagnosis of dysphagia in a HIV$^+$ patient includes
    1. HIV-related stricture
    2. *Candida* esophagitis
    3. *Toxoplasma* esophagitis
    4. herpes simplex esophagitis

210. In the HIV$^+$ individual, common side-effects of trimethoprim/sulfamethoxazole include
    1. granulocytopenia
    2. erythrocytosis
    3. disseminated erythematous rash
    4. thrombocytosis

211. When used for *P. carinii* pneumonia prophylaxis, acceptable dosing regimens for aerosolized pentamidine include
    1. 500 mg every month
    2. 150 mg every month
    3. 1,000 mg every month
    4. 300 mg every month

212. Which of the following antiretroviral and/or immunomodulating agents are undergoing clinical trials as therapy for HIV and/or AIDS?
    1. Interferon-beta
    2. Dideoxyinosine (ddI)
    3. Dideoxycytidine (ddC)
    4. Zidovudine (AZT)

213. Appropriate uses of the HIV-1 antigen (p24 antigen) include
1. monitoring side-effects of antiretroviral therapy
2. monitoring effectiveness of antiviral therapy
3. used to initiate antiretroviral therapy
4. used to predict disease progression (by the reappearance of p24 in serum)

214. Antibodies to HIV-1 are commonly detected by which of the following test(s)?
1. HIV-1 enzyme immunoassay (EIA)
2. Serum for p24
3. Western blot
4. HIV-1 cell culture

215. A 26-year-old hispanic male presents in the clinic complaining of a mucopurulent urethral discharge. He is uncircumcised and has had frequent heterosexual contacts over the last three months. Which of the following organisms should be considered as a cause(s) for this discharge?
1. *N. gonorrhoeae*
2. *C. trachomatis*
3. *Candida albicans*
4. *Toxoplasma gondii*

216. Which of the following may increase the frequency of developing pneumonia?
1. Alcoholism
2. Chronic obstructive pulmonary disease (COPD)
3. Congestive heart failure (CHF)
4. Diabetes mellitus

217. Which of the following are common clinical manifestations of *M. tuberculosis* in the HIV-infected individual?
1. Lymph node disease
2. Lower lobe involvement in the lung
3. Noncavitary pulmonary involvement
4. Bone marrow involvement

Directions Summarized				
A	**B**	**C**	**D**	**E**
1,2,3	1,3	2,4	4	All are
only	only	only	only	correct

218. Management of *M. tuberculosis* in the HIV$^+$ individual may include which of the following?
  1. Isoniazid and rifampin
  2. Ethambutol and pyrazinamide
  3. Streptomycin
  4. Prolonged and possibly indefinite treatment with antituberculosis drugs

219. Viral hepatitis can be caused by which of the following agents?
  1. Hepatitis A
  2. Hepatitis B
  3. Hepatitis delta
  4. Enteric non-A, non-B virus

220. Secondary syphilis can present with which of the following manifestations?
  1. Condyloma lata
  2. Fever of unknown origin
  3. Macular rash
  4. Genital chancre

221. Key psychosocial issues that should be addressed in the management of individuals with HIV-1 include
  1. deteriorating health
  2. treatment options
  3. financial insecurity
  4. prospect of death

222. Cancer commonly arises from tissue that has a self-renewing system, including
  1. colon tissue
  2. breast glands
  3. testicular glands
  4. alveoli

223. Clinical presentations of breast cancer can include
   1. retraction of the nipple
   2. edema of breast tissue
   3. nipple discharge
   4. painless breast lump

224. Factors that prohibit surgery as a possibility for a cure in nonsmall cell carcinoma of the lung include
   1. FEV_1 less than 1.0 liter
   2. CO_2 retention
   3. diagnosis of angina pectoris
   4. history of essential hypertension

DIRECTIONS (Questions 225–240): Each of the questions or incomplete statements below is followed by four or five suggested answers or completions. Select the **one** that is best in each case.

---

225. The **MAJOR** prognostic determinate(s) of individuals diagnosed with cancer include
   A. extent of disease at the time of diagnosis
   B. histologic type and grade/stage of tumor
   C. origin of the tumor
   D. A and B only
   E. A, B, and C

226. Treatment options for individuals with stage I breast cancer include which of the following?
   A. Radiation therapy
   B. Surgical resection
   C. Both
   D. Neither

227. Which of the following has **NOT** been known to transmit HIV-1?
   A. Plasma
   B. Semen
   C. Feces
   D. Whole blood

228. All of the following are the usual modes of HIV-1 transmission **EXCEPT**
A. casual contact
B. parenteral exposure to blood or blood products
C. perinatally from mothers to their infants
D. sexual contact

229. Using the CDC classification system, HIV$^+$ group I is defined as
A. full blown AIDS
B. initial infection with HIV-1 and without symptoms
C. initial infection with HIV-1 and associated lymphadenopathy
D. initial infection with HIV-1 and mononucleosis-like syndrome

230. HIV-1 testing is recommended in all of the following populations **EXCEPT**
A. individuals in mutually monogamous relationships
B. IV-drug users
C. persons who seek treatment for sexually transmitted diseases (STDs)
D. prostitutes

231. All of the following are unique to retroviruses **EXCEPT**
A. genetic transfer of information from DNA to RNA
B. latency period measured in months to years
C. lymphocyte tropism (selective depletion)
D. presence of reverse transcriptase

232. To obtain the definitive diagnosis of *P. carinii* pneumonia, what diagnostic test is commonly used?
A. Fiberoptic bronchoscopy with bronchoalveolar lavage
B. Nonbronchoscopic pulmonary lavage
C. Open lung biopsy
D. Ventilation/perfusion lung scan

233. All of the following are usually associated with HIV-impaired immunity **EXCEPT**
A. allergic rhinitis
B. herpes zoster
C. herpes genitalis
D. tuberculosis

234. The **MOST** common cause of visual loss in the AIDS patient is caused by
   A. *Cryptococcus neoformans*
   B. cytomegalovirus
   C. *Mycobacterium avium-intracellulare*
   D. *M. tuberculosis*

235. A 31-year-old white male presents with a seven-day history of slurred speech, impaired coordination, the inability to urinate, and fevers as high 104 °F. The social history is remarkable for homosexuality and the use of intravenous drugs. All of the following should be included in your differential diagnosis **EXCEPT**
   A. AIDS dementia complex
   B. cryptococcal meningitis
   C. herpes encephalitis
   D. *Toxoplasma* encephalitis

236. A common side-effect of aerosolized pentamidine includes
   A. azotemia
   B. bronchospasm
   C. hypotension
   D. leukopenia

237. In patients with the epidemic form of Kaposi's sarcoma, all of the following are predictors of an indolent course **EXCEPT**
   A. absolute T4 count >400/mm^3
   B. detectable p24 antigen level in serum
   C. few lesions (<25)
   D. no visceral involvement

238. In the HIV-1 infected individual, which of the following diagnostic and/or laboratory tests are indicated initially when focal neurologic symptomatology is present?
   A. Brain biopsy
   B. Computerized tomography of the brain
   C. Lumbar puncture
   D. Pneumoencephalogram

239. All of the following are important defense mechanisms in the prevention of respiratory infections **EXCEPT**
   A. cell mediated immunity
   B. cough reflex
   C. dehumidification of inspired air
   D. filtration of inspired air in the upper airways

240. In *M. tuberculosis,* which of the following represents a more contagious individual?
   A. Individual with a positive AFB smear
   B. Individual with a positive AFB sputum culture
   C. Individual with a positive blood culture for *M. tuberculosis*
   D. Individual with apical infiltrates on a chest x-ray

Explanatory Answers

191. A. Kaposi's sarcoma (KS) lesions in the AIDS patient may present initially as nonpainful pigmented lesions (usually purple or pink), but may be nonpigmented as well. Many areas may be involved, including the skin and extremities, gastrointestinal tract, oral cavity, and the pulmonary parenchyma. Since KS is considered to be an endothelial neoplasm with origins in either capillaries or the lymphatic system, signs of lymphatic obstruction may also be present. (Ref. 12, pp. 1080–1081)

192. A. The Centers for Disease Control (CDC) developed the AIDS case definition in 1982, and it is defined as the occurrence of a disease that is indicative of underlying cellular immunodeficiency in a person without a condition known to be associated with an increased incidence of diseases related to cellular immunodeficiency. While candidiasis, KS, *P. carinii*, and pulmonary *M. tuberculosis* can all occur with a cellular immunodeficiency, pulmonary *M. tuberculosis* can also occur in the normal host. (Ref. 12, pp. 1059–1060)

193. B. Human immunodeficiency virus type-1 (HIV-1) is the etiologic agent that causes AIDS and has a selective tropism for the T4 helper cell. Since the T4 cell is involved in all immune responses, a decrease like the one seen in the HIV-1 infection and AIDS would cause multiple immunologic abnormalities. Hence, B cell abnormalities and decreased parasite killing would occur. Increased response to soluble antigen and chemotaxis would most likely occur if the immune system remained intact. (Ref. 12, pp. 1046–1059)

194. E. Diseases associated with the pulmonary system are the most common in individuals infected with HIV-1. High fevers and shortness of breath are typical symptoms of *P. carinii* and CMV pneumonitis. A dry cough is usually present as well, but not always. Pulmonary tuberculosis and viral pneumonia need to be considered in the differential as well. Tuberculosis is of particular concern because of the growing number of cases that are diagnosed in the HIV-1 infected individual. (Ref. 13, p. 26)

195. C. *P. carinii* and CMV pneumonia usually cause a characteristic diffuse interstitial pattern on the chest radiograph. Pulmonary tuberculosis usually presents with apical infiltrates and *S. pneumoniae* causes lobar consolidation. (Ref. 14, p. 20)

196. C. Kaposi's sarcoma lesions can occur anywhere, but are most common in the skin and viscera. (Ref. 12, pp. 1080–1081)

197. B. The goal of the HIV-1 evaluation should include evaluation of the immune system, classification of the HIV infection using the CDC classification system, identification and treatment of infectious and neoplastic complications, institution of approved antiretroviral therapy, and identification of patients who may benefit from experimental therapeutics. (Ref. 13, p. 24)

198. E. To date, zidovudine is indicated in individuals who have T4 levels that are less than $500/mm^3$, regardless of symptoms. Recent evidence suggests that early evaluation of individuals infected with HIV-1 may be of increased benefit through earlier identification and treatment with antiviral drugs. Zidovudine has been demonstrated in National Institute of Health trials to have a statistically significant benefit when compared to a placebo in patients with symptomatic or asymptomatic HIV-1 infection. Caution should be used when prescribing zidovudine, since the long-term benefits and side-effects in these individuals are still undetermined. (Refs. 15, pp. 727–737; 16, pp. 941–949)

199. A. A thorough history is the most important aspect of the evaluation of a patient infected with HIV-1. It is essential to identify and distinguish HIV-related conditions from other findings. The focus should be on HIV risk factors, medical history (especially a history of STDs), and a comprehensive review of the system. Although, it is important to know about past immunizations, this particular information should not be sought out initially. (Ref. 13, p. 25)

200. E. Collectively, pulmonary complications account for the greatest portion of morbidity and mortality in AIDS patients. *P. carinii* is the most common AIDS-related infection. Other opportunistic pulmonary infections can be caused by cytomegalovirus, tuberculosis, atypical mycobacteriosis, histoplasmosis, cryptococcosis, and coccidioidomycosis. Neoplasms and lymphoproliferative disorders such as lymphoma, Kaposi's sarcoma, and lympoid interstitial pneumonitis can also cause pulmonary complications. (Ref. 13, p. 31)

201. A. Brainstem lymphoma, cryptococcal meningitis, and *Toxoplasma* encephalitis all could occur acutely and have the characteristic signs and symptoms of dizziness, weakness, fevers, and headaches. AIDS dementia complex (ADC) may also have the same signs and symptoms, but usually presents as a slowly progressive disease without focal findings. (Ref. 13, pp. 28–31)

202. B. The absolute T4 (also referred to as OKT4+ or CD4+) cell count is the main measure of immune compromise secondary to HIV-1 infection. Further assessment of immune function involves determination of serum beta-2-microglobulin. The absolute T4 count reflects the activity of the HIV-1 infection, and, in concert with beta-2-microglobulin, is predictive of the risk of clinical disease progression. With advanced HIV-1 infection, one would expect a decreased T4 count and an elevated beta-2-microglobulin. (Ref. 14, p. 20)

203. C. Sulfadiazine and pyrimethamine are the two drugs that seem to be most effective against *Toxoplasma* encephalitis. Clindamycin plus pyrimethamine can be used as an alternative for those individuals allergic to sulfa drugs. Dapsone, trimetrexate, and spiramycin are also being assessed. (Ref. 12, p. 1107)

204. E. Oral candidiasis will respond to either topical therapy, such as nystatin and clotrimazole, or systemic therapy, like ketoconazole and fluconazole. (Ref. 12, p. 1108)

205. E. Zidovudine causes many side-effects. Among the most common are anemia, macrocytosis, nausea, and headaches. (Ref. 12, pp. 1103–1104)

206. A. Trimethoprim/sulfamethoxazole, trimethoprim-dapsone, and pentamidine isethionate may be used to treat *P. carinii* pneumonia. Trimethoprim/sulfamethoxazole is the drug of choice for nonallergic individuals, since it can be given orally and can possibly shorten or eliminate hospitalizations. (Ref. 12, pp. 1104–1107)

207. B. Individuals who have symptomatic HIV infection should have serology drawn for CMV, EBV, and HSV. These viruses may cause symptomatic disease following activation. They may also adversely affect cell-mediated immunity, and augment the HIV infection itself. *Toxoplasma* can be another useful baseline study. Disease caused by this intracellular parasite occurs mainly through reactivation of a prior infection. The immune-compromised host most often develops encephalitis or abscesses; retinitis or pneumonitis are less common forms. The absolute T4 count is the main measure of immune compromise secondary to HIV. T4 levels are used to determine whether antiretroviral therapy will be given. For example, standard protocols call for therapy with zidovudine (AZT) to begin only when there is evidence of immune compromise (CD4$^+$ levels 500/mm^3). (Ref. 14, p. 20)

208. B.   The treatment of choice for cryptococcal meningitis is amphotericin B. Fluconazole has been approved for the treatment of acute cryptococcal meningitis as well. Fluconazole can be given orally and intravenously, which may shorten hospitalizations and eliminate the use of venous catheters. (Ref. 12, p. 1109)

209. C.   *Candida* and herpes simplex are two agents that may cause dysphagia and esophagitis in an HIV$^+$ patient. Other possible causes of esophageal pathology include zidovudine therapy, lymphoma, and Kaposi's sarcoma. (Refs. 12, p. 1069; 13, p. 26)

210. B.   Individuals infected with HIV and receiving trimethoprim/sulfamethoxazole may have erythematous skin rashes, granulocytopenia, elevations in liver enzymes, abnormalities in kidney function due to nephritis, and nausea and vomiting. These adverse reactions seem to be more prevalent in the HIV population and can occur in 50% to 100% of patients with AIDS. The exact reason for this is still unclear. (Ref. 12, p. 1105)

211. D.   An effective regimen for the prophylactic treatment of *P. carinii* pneumonia is aerosolized pentamidine 300 mg every month. Bactrim (trimethoprim/sulfamethoxazole) is another drug that has been determined to be effective for prophylaxis. Other potential agents include dapsone plus trimethoprim and pyrimethamine plus sulfadoxine. (Refs. 12, p. 1107; 17, pp. 54–69)

212. E.   Interferon-beta, ddI, ddC, and zidovudine are all agents that are undergoing clinical evaluation. Zidovudine has already been approved by the Food and Drug Administration for individuals with CD4 levels less than 500/mm^3. However, zidovudine continues to be studied in combination with other drugs, like acyclovir, or in comparative studies with drugs like ddC. Dideoxyinosine (ddI) recently has been approved for individuals who either are intolerant to zidovudine therapy or begin to deteriorate while receiving zidovudine. (Ref. 12, p. 1102)

213. C. Uses for the p24 antigen include detection of HIV-1 in cell culture, prediction of disease progression, monitoring antiviral therapy, and evaluating the HIV-1 infection of newborns. (Ref. 12, p. 1098)

214. B. Human immunodeficiency virus type 1 (HIV-1) enzyme immunoassay (EIA) and the Western blot are proven methods to determine the presence of antibodies against HIV-1. (Ref. 12, p. 1092)

215. A. *N. gonorrhoeae, C. trachomatis,* and *C. albicans* are all possible causes for urethritis in the male. *C. albicans* usually is not considered initially, but in uncircumcised individuals it is a possibility. (Ref. 12, pp. 942–952)

216. E. Individuals with alcoholism, COPD, CHF, and diabetes mellitus have been noted to have an increased frequency of pneumonia. For example, alcoholics are likely to develop pneumonia caused by anaerobic bacteria, whereas individuals with COPD may develop pneumonia caused by *S. pneumoniae* and *Haemophilus influenzae.* (Ref. 12, pp. 541–542)

217. E. Extrapulmonary involvement of *M. tuberculosis* occurs in as many as 50% of individuals who are HIV⁺ and have contracted the organism. Common manifestations include lymph node involvement, lower lobe involvement of the lung, noncavitary pulmonary involvement, and bone marrow disease. (Ref. 12, p. 1886)

218. E. Prolonged and possibly indefinite treatment of tuberculosis in the HIV⁺ patient is necessary to prevent relapse and further dissemination. Appropriate drugs include isoniazid, rifampin, ethambutol, pyrazinamide, and streptomycin. A common combination of drugs given for active tuberculosis include isoniazid, rifampin, and ethambutol. (Ref. 12, p. 1109)

219. E. Acute viral hepatitis can be caused by five viral agents: hepatitis A, hepatitis B, hepatitis delta, parenteral non-A, non-B, and enteric non-A, non-B. Recently, non-A, non-B viruses have been renamed as hepatitis C. (Ref. 12, p. 1001)

220. E. Secondary syphilis often causes disseminated manifestations that are commonly seen in the skin, mouth and throat, genitalia, and central nervous system. Less common manifestations can occur in the renal and gastrointestinal systems. Thus, lesions like condyloma lata can be seen, as well as the presence of fevers, rashes, and genital chancres. (Ref. 12, pp. 1797–1799)

221. E. Patients diagnosed in any group or stage of the HIV-1 infection may develop psychosocial problems, apart from physical illness. Fear and uncertainty play a key role in these problems. Patients may face deteriorating health, decisions about treatment, job loss and financial insecurity, loss of emotional support, problems with relationships, changes in lifestyle and the prospect of death. The clinician must be extremely sensitive to these issues, and must be able to identify sources of available support. (Ref. 14, p. 21)

222. A. Cancer commonly arises in organs that have a self-renewing system. Colon tissue, breast, and testicular glands, the epithelium of the bronchial tree, are some examples of this phenomenon. (Ref. 18, p. 369)

223. E. Most individuals present with a painless breast lump when first diagnosed with breast cancer. Edema of the breast tissue, retraction of the nipple, and nipple discharge can also occur, but they usually indicate advanced disease. (Ref. 18, p. 441)

224. A. It is imperative to fully evaluate a patient with resectable non-small cell lung cancer prior to surgery. Coexisting medical conditions such as angina pectoris is a contraindication to surgery. Other contraindications include CO_2 retention, poor pulmonary function (FEV_1 less than 1.0 liter) and a diagnosis of pulmonary hypertension. (Ref. 18, pp. 446–447)

225. E. Once diagnosed with malignant tumors, the prognosis can be somewhat determined by the extent of the disease at the time of diagnosis, histologic type and grade/stage of tumor, and the origin of the tumor. Individuals with localized noninvasive tumors will generally do better than individuals with metastatic and locally aggressive tumors. (Ref. 18, p. 381)

226. C. Treatment options for stage I breast cancer may include surgical resection (mastectomy) or excision of the primary tumor with radiation therapy. The axillary lymph nodes should be dissected at the time of surgery to determine whether adjuvant chemotherapy is necessary to prevent recurrence. (Ref. 18, p. 442)

227. C. HIV has only been isolated from blood and blood products, semen, vaginal secretions, the uterine cervix, saliva, breast milk, tears, urine, cerebrospinal fluid, alveolar fluid, and amniotic fluid. HIV is widely accepted to be transmitted through blood, blood products, and semen. Feces has not been known to transmit the virus, although universal precautions should be adhered to with all body fluids and products. (Ref. 12, p. 1038)

228. A. HIV-1 is transmitted almost exclusively through sexual contact, parenteral exposure to blood or blood products, and perinatally from infected mothers to their infants. There have not been any cases linked to casual contact such as hugging or kissing. (Ref. 12, pp. 1036–1038)

229. D. According to the CDC, HIV$^+$ group I is defined as an acute illness with a documented mononucleosis-like syndrome. Group II corresponds with an asymptomatic infection, group III is associated with persistent generalized lymphadenopathy (PGL), and group IV is full blown AIDS (ie, the presence of AIDS indicator disease *P. carinii* pneumonia). (Ref. 12, p. 103)

230. A. The U.S. Public Health Service recommends that any individual who has exposure to body fluids or products either through sexual activity, parenterally, or perinatally should be counseled and tested for HIV-1. They also recommend counseling and testing for the following groups: persons anticipating marriage; persons who have prolonged diarrhea, lympadenopathy, fevers, or weight loss; persons diagnosed with tuberculosis, herpes, and candidiasis; persons in correctional institutions; persons who have had contact with the above. (Ref. 12, pp. 1041–1042)

231. A. A retrovirus has the ability to transcribe its genetic information from the virion RNA into DNA. This process is aided by the enzyme, reverse transcriptase. Research has been directed toward the inhibition of reverse transcriptase in the hopes of slowing the replication process of the virus. Zidovudine, a nucleoside analogue, has already been proven to be effective; other similar drugs, such as ddI and ddC, are presently undergoing clinical evaluation. (Ref. 12, pp. 1046–1047)

232. A. While nonbronchoscopic pulmonary lavage, open lung biopsy, and ventilation/perfusion lung scan may all be used to diagnose *P. carinii* pneumonia, fiberoptic bronchoscopy with bronchoalveolar lavage remains the most common and reliable method of diagnosis. The diagnosis of pneumocystis usually can be established by bronchoscopy in over 90% of AIDS patients. (Ref. 12, p. 2106)

233. A. Herpes zoster, herpes genitalis, and tuberculosis can occur with impaired immunity, whereas allergic rhinitis usually does not. A history of recurrent or unusual infections may also suggest impaired immunity. (Ref. 13, pp. 25–26)

234. B. Cytomegalovirus is by far the most common cause of retinitis and subsequent vision loss in the AIDS patient. Other less common causes of ocular pathology and possible vision loss include toxoplasmosis, herpes, *Cryptococcus, Candida, M. avium-intracellulare,* and tuberculosis. (Ref. 13, p. 28)

235. A. Cryptococcal meningitis, herpes encephalitis, and *Toxoplasma* encephalitis are all possibilities that should be included in the differential. AIDS dementia complex usually presents in a slowly progressive manner,

Figure 1

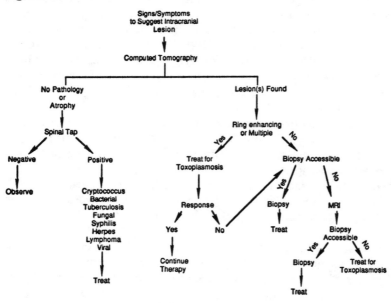

rather than acutely; therefore, it would not be included in the differential. (Ref. 13, pp. 28–29)

236. B. Aerosolized pentamidine has little systemic effect, since the drug is not readily absorbed into the bloodstream from the lungs. However, bronchospasms seem to be very common, but are easily treated with bronchodilators. (Ref. 12, p. 110)

237. B. In the epidemic form of Kaposis's sarcoma, prognostic variables that may predict an indolent course include: few lesions, decreased growth rate of lesions, no visceral involvement, no constitutional symptoms (fevers, night sweats, or weight loss), no history of opportunistic infections, T4 count that is greater than 400 mm^3, normal sedimentation rate, nondetectable p24 levels in the serum, a normal beta-2-microglobulin, and a normal complete blood count (CBC). In contrast, an aggressive course may be predicted if the exact opposite of the above were to occur, with minor exceptions, of course. (Ref. 12, p. 1081)

238. B. Computerized imaging of the brain (CT) is the first diagnostic test that should be done to rule out intracranial lesions. The algorithm in Figure 1 may be of use when evaluating patients with neurologic signs and symptoms. (Ref. 12, p. 1077)

239. C. Filtration and humidification of inspired air, cough reflex, tracheobronchial secretions, cell mediated and humoral immunity, and the presence of polymorphonuclear neutrophils are all important mechanisms that help prevent respiratory infections. (Ref. 12, p. 541)

240. A. In general, individuals who have a positive sputum smear for AFB are likely to be more contagious than individuals with apical infiltrates on the chest x-ray, or positive cultures. (Ref. 12, p. 1880)

7 Surgery

241. The **MOST** common complication following appendectomy is
    A. fecal fistula
    B. retained foreign body
    C. pylephlebitis
    D. wound infection

242. The single therapeutic modality capable of curing a large percentage of stage I breast cancer lesions is
    A. hormonal therapy
    B. multiple agent chemotherapy
    C. radiotherapy
    D. surgery

243. The chief complaint of females subsequently diagnosed with breast cancer is
    A. breast dimpling
    B. breast mass
    C. breast pain
    D. nipple discharge

244. The MOST important means of wound healing in healing by primary intention is from which of the following mechanisms?
   A. Accurate surgical closure
   B. Contraction
   C. Epithelialization
   D. Hypertrophic scarring

245. The suture material that is the strongest and least reactive to tissue is
   A. catgut
   B. chromic
   C. nylon
   D. silk
   E. stainless steel

246. In otherwise healthy patients who are scheduled for elective surgery, which preoperative screening tests should be routinely performed?
   A. Partial thromboplastin time (PTT)
   B. Prothrombin time (PT)
   C. Both
   D. Neither

247. The fluid of choice for rapid volume replacement for treatment of hypovolemic shock is
   A. albumin
   B. 5% dextrose in water
   C. normal saline
   D. Ringer's lactate

248. A patient with a hand wound which occurred three days ago is seen in the emergency department with a 1-cm wide × 0.5-cm deep circular wound on the thenar eminence. Evidence of red streaking is seen on the volar surface of the forearm. What additional physical exam finding would be MOST likely?
   A. Crepitus
   B. Fever
   C. Lymph node enlargement
   D. Petechiae

249. Which intraabdominal organ is **MOST** susceptible to rupture by trauma?
A. Colon
B. Liver
C. Spleen
D. Stomach
E. Urinary bladder

250. The goal of the workup of the patient with an acute abdominal complaint is to
A. administer analgesics in cases of severe pain as soon as the patient is seen, so that suffering can be eliminated during the workup
B. diagnose the patient within 15 to 30 minutes so that definitive treatment can be given
C. observe the patient's symptom development over 8 to 10 hours for signs of change of symptoms
D. depend on lab and diagnostic test results to make the diagnosis

251. The pathogenesis of deep vein thrombosis is attributed to all of the following **EXCEPT**
A. endothelial injury
B. hypercoagulability
C. inflammation
D. stasis

252. The **MOST** likely cause of fever in the first 24 hours after an operation is
A. atelectasis
B. drug fever
C. thrombophlebitis
D. urinary tract infection
E. wound infection

253. The **MOST** common form of breast cancer is
A. comedocarcinoma
B. fibroadenoma
C. infiltrating ductal carcinoma
D. infiltrating lobular carcinoma
E. Paget's disease

254. The pain of cholecystitis is commonly referred to what area of the body?
   A. Chest
   B. Neck
   C. Perineum
   D. Scapula tip
   E. Umbilicus

255. The appropriate treatment for sigmoid volvulus is
   A. barium enema
   B. decompression with a soft rubber tube via sigmoidoscopy
   C. detorsion by operative procedure through an abdominal incision
   D. sigmoid resection

256. The **MOST** common cause of paralytic ileus is
   A. abdominal operation
   B. hemorrhage
   C. infection
   D. trauma to retroperitoneal nerves
   E. spinal cord lesions

257. Radiographic evidence of dilated small and large intestine with gas scattered diffusely throughout the intestinal tract is consistent with
   A. mechanical bowel obstruction
   B. paralytic ileus
   C. both
   D. neither

258. Wound dehiscence usually occurs during which of the following postoperative timeframes?
   A. 1 to 2 days
   B. 5 to 7 days
   C. 8 to 9 days
   D. Six weeks
   E. Three months

259. The benefit of short-term smoking cessation preoperatively is
  A. an increased vital capacity
  B. an interruption of normal mucociliary functioning
  C. a decreased chance of spread of infection through the intubation process
  D. a decreased level of blood carbon monoxide
  E. a decreased rate of bronchospastic problems with anesthesia induction

260. Most patients who have normal erythrocytes will have adequate oxygen delivery if the hematocrit is at **LEAST**
  A. 10%
  B. 15%
  C. 20%
  D. 25%
  E. 30%

261. Which of the following treatments are appropriate to reverse the effects of heparin preoperatively?
  A. Fresh frozen plasma
  B. Protamine
  C. Vitamin C
  D. Vitamin K

262. Although heparin affects all coagulation tests, the **MOST** sensitive test is considered to be
  A. activated partial thromboplastin time (PTT)
  B. bleeding time
  C. platelet count
  D. platelet function
  E. prothrombin time (PT)

263. Which of the following is considered to be the **LEAST** precise measurement of protein stores of the surgical patient?
  A. Absolute lymphocyte count
  B. Delayed cutaneous hypersensitivity
  C. Midarm muscle circumference
  D. Serum albumin
  E. Serum transferrin

264. An adult patient has a burn on the leg resulting from the spill of a pot of coffee. The wound on the upper and lower right leg is bright red and has various sized bullae which are moist and weeping. The burns are thickened by edema, but remain pliable. The burns are hypersensitive. This burn could be characterized as

A. first-degree
B. superficial second-degree
C. deep dermal second-degree
D. full thickness or third-degree

265. Which of the following is **NOT** a universal criteria for organ donation?

A. The donor must be free from active infections
B. The donor must have no history of previous communicable disease
C. The donor organs must be free of previous disease
D. The donor and recipient must be of compatible weight and body build

266. A patient receives a blow to the head and has a brief period of unconsciousness. The patient then awakens and has no neurologic deficits. The patient then has a gradual deterioration of consciousness that progresses to coma and possibly death. This scenario is compatible with which diagnosis?

A. Epidural hematoma
B. Primary brain injury
C. Skull fracture
D. Spinal cord injury
E. Subdural hematoma

267. Lumbar disc herniation is treated acutely with all of the following **EXCEPT**

A. analgesics
B. bed rest
C. local heat
D. muscle relaxants
E. physical therapy

268. In the United States, the **MOST** common type of renal calculi are composed of
   A. calcium
   B. cystine
   C. struvite
   D. uric acid

269. The **MOST** common etiology of congenital heart disease is
   A. atrial septal defect
   B. coarctation of the aorta
   C. tetralogy of Fallot
   D. transposition of the great vessels
   E. ventricular septal defect

270. Treatment for pulmonary embolism should begin with
   A. anticoagulant therapy using sodium warfarin
   B. embolectomy
   C. placement of a vena cava filter
   D. rapid diagnosis of the problem

271. Asymptomatic abdominal aortic aneurysms are to be resected and replaced with a graft when they reach what size?
   A. 4 cm
   B. 5 cm
   C. 6 cm
   D. 7 cm
   E. 8 cm

272. Splenectomy is usually indicated in patients with
   A. acquired chemical-induced hemolytic anemia
   B. glucose 6-phosphate dehydrogenase (G-6-PD) deficiency
   C. hereditary elliptocytosis
   D. hereditary spherocytosis
   E. sickle cell anemia

273. An enlargement in the anterior auricular lymph nodes is associated with
   A. conjunctiva and eyelid infection
   B. dental infection
   C. oral cavity or pharyngeal infection
   D. scalp infection
   E. tuberculosis

274. All of the following are true about pilonidal cysts **EXCEPT** they
   A. occur commonly in the sacrococcygeal area
   B. may occur in the axilla, umbilicus, beard region, and interdigital web spaces of the hands or feet
   C. occur more often in men than women; young than old
   D. are due mostly to the foreign body effect of the penetration of the skin by hair
   E. are managed surgically, usually with incision and drainage, and antibiotics

275. Which of the following is **FALSE** concerning solitary thyroid nodules?
   A. Hyperfunctioning (hot) nodules are often malignant
   B. The main objective in evaluating the nodule is to detect malignancy
   C. Many etiologies can be suppressed with administration of T4
   D. Most thyroid nodules are benign and do not require surgical resection

276. Which of the following patients with traumatic splenic rupture should routinely be candidates for splenectomy?
   A. Adults
   B. Children
   C. Both
   D. Neither

277. Dull, aching constant left lower quadrant pain in a 72-year-old patient would **MOST** likely be associated with
   A. appendicitis
   B. colon cancer
   C. diverticulitis
   D. urinary tract infection
   E. volvulus

278. All of the following describe a benign adnexal mass **EXCEPT**
- **A.** bilateral
- **B.** cystic
- **C.** mobile
- **D.** size <10 cm
- **E.** smooth

279. The **MOST** common complication of acute pancreatitis is pancreatic
- **A.** abscess
- **B.** cellulitis
- **C.** fistula
- **D.** pseudocyst

280. In patients with transient ischemic attacks, the treatment of choice is
- **A.** antiplatelet agents
- **B.** carotid endarterectomy
- **C.** cholesterol-lowering agents
- **D.** vasodilators

281. Degenerative disc disease is **MOST** common in which spinal region?
- **A.** Cervical
- **B.** Lumbar
- **C.** Thoracic
- **D.** Sacral

282. The age at which all women should be screened by annual mammography is
- **A.** 30
- **B.** 40
- **C.** 50
- **D.** 60

283. In documenting the size of a mass, which of the following is **CORRECT?**
- **A.** An abdominal mass measuring two fingers by three fingers
- **B.** A grapefruit-sized enlargement of the uterus
- **C.** A 1-in × $^1/_2$-in mass attached to the spermatic cord
- **D.** A pea-sized lump in the breast
- **E.** A 0.5-cm diameter round mass attached to the tendon

284. Primary treatment of amebic liver abscess includes
  A. amebicidal drug, ie, metronidazole
  B. percutaneous aspiration of the abscess
  C. both choice A and choice B
  D. neither choice A nor choice B

285. For patients with adequately controlled seizures, which of the following would be appropriate?
  A. Cancel any surgical procedure permanently
  B. Discontinue anticonvulsant therapy the night before surgery
  C. Manage uremia, hypernatremia, and hyponatremia carefully during the perioperative period, since these conditions predispose to seizures
  D. Refer the patient to a neurologist who will determine if the patient is able to be cleared for surgery

286. Physical findings associated with testicular torsion include
  A. mild pain in the testicle is elicited upon palpation
  B. pain is relieved upon elevation of the scrotum
  C. the affected testicle is in the transverse position
  D. the affected testicle is usually lower in the scrotum than the unaffected testicle

287. Whether using the Parkland or modified Brooke formula for fluid resuscitation in the severely burned patient, what proportion of the fluid should be administered during the first eight hours?
  A. $^1/_5$
  B. $^1/_4$
  C. $^1/_3$
  D. $^1/_2$
  E. $^2/_3$

288. Using the rule of nines, an adult who has burns over the right anterior arm and right anterior leg would have approximately what percentage of his body burned?
  A. 6%
  B. 13.5%
  C. 18.5%
  D. 27%

289. Which of the following are considered appropriate treatments for anorectal abscesses?
   A. Treatment of any underlying cause, ie, carcinoma, tuberculosis, or colitis, should be instituted
   B. Prompt incision and drainage is performed, even if the mass is not yet fluctuant
   C. Both
   D. Neither

290. A thrill that is palpated over an artery throughout the cardiac cycle is associated with
   A. arteriovenous fistula
   B. severe stenosis
   C. both choice A and choice B
   D. neither choice A nor choice B

291. Positive estrogen receptor assay of a breast tumor is associated with
   A. the degree of differentiation of the tumor
   B. the efficacy of hormonal manipulation
   C. the extent of lymph node involvement
   D. the need for cancer chemotherapy

292. The goal of the perioperative care of the diabetic surgical patient is to maintain a state of mild hyperglycemia in order to avoid hypoglycemia. At what level of blood glucose would additional insulin treatment be required?
   A. 100 mg/dL
   B. 150 mg/dL
   C. 200 mg/dL
   D. 250 mg/dL
   E. 300 mg/dL

DIRECTIONS (Questions 293–325): For each of the questions or incomplete statements below, **one or more** of the answers or completions given are correct. Select:

- A   if only **1, 2,** and **3** are correct,
- B   if only **1** and **3** are correct,
- C   if only **2** and **4** are correct,
- D   if only **4** is correct,
- E   if **all** are correct.

293. In a patient with breast cancer, a poor prognosis is indicated by
    1. mass with fixation to underlying structures
    2. peau d'orange (orange peel skin)
    3. cancer in a supraclavicular lymph node
    4. hypercalcemia

294. Guidelines for treatment of tetanus-prone wounds in the patient immunized over ten years ago include which of the following?
    1. Intramuscular administration of 0.5 mL of tetanus toxoid
    2. Intramuscular administration of 250 units of tetanus immune globulin
    3. Careful debridement and copious irrigation of the wound
    4. Intravenous administration of penicillin

295. It is important to drain wounds when abnormal fluid collections are expected to form because the fluid collection may be associated with
    1. bacterial growth
    2. tissue irritation or necrosis
    3. loss of vascularity
    4. pressure on adjacent organs

296. Items of importance in the surgical history that may indicate perioperative bleeding problems include
    1. aspirin therapy within the previous week
    2. current dietary intake
    3. recent history of binge drinking
    4. current antibiotic therapy

Directions Summarized				
A	**B**	**C**	**D**	**E**
1,2,3	1,3	2,4	4	All are
only	only	only	only	correct

297. A 50-year-old patient is diagnosed with cellulitis of the left lower leg. Which of the following treatments is/are considered appropriate?
   1. Warm soaks
   2. Elevation of the leg
   3. High-dose penicillin
   4. Range of motion exercises

298. The majority of cases of acute pancreatitis in the United States are associated with which of the following conditions?
   1. Trauma
   2. Gallstones
   3. Carcinoma
   4. Alcoholism

299. In establishing the diagnosis of acute appendicitis, which of the following usually occurs?
   1. Pain develops prior to the onset of vomiting
   2. Fever up to 103° to 104° prior to the development of pain
   3. Abdominal tenderness, although variable in location and intensity, must be demonstrated somewhere in the abdomen
   4. Testicular referred pain develops

300. A 67-year-old male patient presents with swelling and a dull, aching pain in the groin. A protrusion is felt on the finger pad of the examining finger during the hernia examination. No mass is felt in the scrotum. Which of the following statements would be **CORRECT** about this case?
   1. The patient needs surgery so that the hernia does not incarcerate or strangulate
   2. Anatomically, the hernia arises medial to the inferior deep epigastric artery
   3. He has the most common type of hernia
   4. The etiology of the hernia is most probably wear and tear

301. Patients with hiatal hernias are usually treated medically for their symptoms. What conditions would make surgery necessary?
   1. Unwillingness of the patient to lose weight
   2. Ulceration and bleeding
   3. Allergy to H_2 blockers
   4. Enlargement of the hernia

302. Surgery is the definitive treatment for patients with which duodenal ulcer complication(s)?
   1. Severe, persistent, or recurrent bleeding
   2. Gastric outlet obstruction
   3. Perforation of the duodenal wall
   4. Postsurgical recurrence of ulcers

303. Important indicators of nutritional adequacy in surgical patients include
   1. serum albumin
   2. plasma transferrin
   3. triceps skinfold thickness
   4. delayed cutaneous hypersensitivity

304. Factors that increase life-threatening cardiac complications in the postoperative period include
   1. myocardial infarction within the past six months
   2. preoperative S3 gallop
   3. age greater than 70 years
   4. orthopedic operation

305. Common causes of intestinal obstruction in adults include
   1. adhesions
   2. hernias
   3. tumors
   4. intussusception

306. Intestinal obstruction from within the gut occluding the lumen is termed obturation. In the United States, it is frequently caused by
   1. bezoars
   2. gallstone ileus
   3. parasitic infections
   4. fecal impaction

Directions Summarized				
A	**B**	**C**	**D**	**E**
1,2,3	1,3	2,4	4	All are
only	only	only	only	correct

307. Uncomplicated hemorrhoids are characterized by
  1. dull pain
  2. protrusion
  3. bleeding
  4. pruritus

308. Risk factors for postoperative pneumonia include
  1. long preoperative hospitalization period
  2. smoking
  3. long operations
  4. pulmonary edema

309. A patient presents to the emergency room in a coma of unknown origin. After establishing an airway, checking for adequate circulation, and drawing of blood for laboratory studies, which of the following should be given **NEXT**?
  1. Naloxone hydrochloride (Narcan) 0.4 to 0.8 mg IV
  2. Thiamine 100 mg IV
  3. Dextrose 25 to 50 g IV
  4. Broad spectrum antibiotic, loading dose, IV

310. When using epinephrine-containing solutions for infiltrative local anesthesia, consideration should be given to
  1. avoiding body parts with end-terminal arteries, like fingers and toes
  2. using it routinely in contaminated wounds
  3. cautious administration in patients with heart disease or peripheral vascular disease
  4. limiting the total amount of epinephrine injected to no more than 2 mg

311. When thinking about performing elective surgery on a pregnant patient under general anesthesia, considerations would include
   1. avoiding elective operations during the first trimester of pregnancy
   2. risking development of supine hypotension syndrome during the last trimester of pregnancy
   3. categorizing all pregnant patients after 12 weeks gestation as having "full stomachs" because of decreased gastric emptying
   4. performing no special monitoring of the fetus during the operation, just careful monitoring of the mother's vital signs

312. Criteria indicating inoperable thorax tumors include
   1. peripheral location
   2. positive pleural effusion cytology
   3. metastasis limited to hilar nodes
   4. Horner's syndrome

313. Complications of duodenal ulcers for which definitive ulcer surgery is indicated include
   1. intractable pain
   2. acute perforation
   3. gastric outlet obstruction
   4. acute hemorrhage

314. When using the TNM system for classifying breast tumors, which of the following would be considered stage IV?
   1. $T_2 N_1 M_0$
   2. $T_3 N_3 M_0$
   3. $T_1 N_2 M_0$
   4. $T_1 N_1 M_1$

315. Common evidence indicating traumatic injury to the kidneys, ureters, or bladder includes
   1. gross hematuria on inspection of urine
   2. white blood cells on the microscopic examination of urine
   3. trace hematuria on the dipstick examination of urine
   4. increased urine specific gravity

Directions Summarized				
A	**B**	**C**	**D**	**E**
1,2,3	1,3	2,4	4	All are
only	only	only	only	correct

316. Which of the following are **TRUE** statements concerning testicular carcinoma?
1. Most are found in men between 20 and 40 years of age
2. Mixed cell patterns, particularly nonseminomatous tumors, are most common
3. Painless testicular enlargement and heaviness often are presenting complaints
4. Overall survival rates are poor

317. Varicose veins are
1. mostly a cosmetic problem
2. related to venous valvular incompetence
3. treated successfully with elastic stockings, sclerotherapy, or vein stripping
4. often related to the development of large pulmonary emboli

318. Which of the following statements is/are **TRUE** concerning intermittent claudication?
1. Pain may be located in the calf, thigh, or buttocks
2. Pain or tightness is experienced at rest
3. Impotence may be an associated symptom
4. Suggests that vascular disease is limited to the extremity

319. Complications of thyroidectomy include
1. injury to the inferior laryngeal nerves
2. injury to the superior laryngeal nerves
3. hypoparathyroidism
4. wound hemorrhage

320. Biopsied lymph nodes may routinely be sent for which of the following studies?
1. Histology
2. Bacterial cultures
3. Cytology
4. Fungal cultures

321. Which of the following is/are **TRUE** concerning myxomas?
1. They are most likely to be found in the right atrium
2. Patients exhibit symptoms of systemic embolization and have a positional heart murmur
3. Resection usually is not necessary
4. Morbidity and mortality is usually low

322. Findings seen in patients after coronary artery bypass grafting with saphenous vein grafts include
1. reduced angina pain
2. improved ventricular function
3. reduced chance of recurrent myocardial infarction
4. reduced rates of atherosclerosis in the grafts over time

323. Complications of endoscopic spincterotomy as treatment for symptomatic or large (>1 cm) common bile duct stones include
1. bleeding
2. pancreatitis
3. cholangitis
4. duodenal perforation

324. Ways to decrease infection in surgical patients include
1. limiting conversation in the operating room
2. a five-minute initial scrub of operative team hands
3. use of paper drapes
4. shaving hair at the operative site just prior to the operation

325. Preoperative chest roentgenograms would be warranted in which of the following scenarios?
1. A 40-year-old white male with a 20 pack/year smoking history undergoing vagotomy for recurrent peptic ulcer disease
2. A 55-year-old black female with a ten-year history of asthma
3. A 60-year-old black female with 40 pack/year smoking history and mild COPD undergoing a vaginal hysterectomy for bitroids
4. A 36-year-old hispanic male, in good physical health, undergoing inguinal herniorrhaphy

---

DIRECTIONS (Questions 326–340): Each group of lettered headings below is followed by a list of numbered words or phrases. For each numbered word or phrase, select:

 A if the item is associated with **A only,**
 B if the item is associated with **B only,**
 C if the item is associated with **both A and B,**
 D if the item is associated with **neither A nor B.**

Questions 326–328:
 A. Direct inguinal hernia
 B. Indirect inguinal hernia
 C. Both
 D. Neither

326. Arises medial of inferior deep epigastric artery

327. Commonly descends into the scrotum

328. More common in women than in men

Questions 329–331:
 A. Are found in the peripheral lung fields
 B. Are found in the central lung fields
 C. Both
 D. Neither

329. Adenocarcinoma

330. Large cell carcinomas

331. Small cell tumors

Questions 332–335:
    A. Ulcerative colitis
    B. Granulomatous colitis (Crohn's disease)
    C. Both
    D. Neither

332. Increased risk for toxic megacolon

333. Bloody diarrhea

334. Increased risk for colon cancer

335. Barium enema demonstrates "skip areas"

Questions 336–338: Match the correct mediastinal tumor to the systemic syndrome caused by ectopic hormone production.
    A. Pheochromocytoma
    B. Carcinoid
    C. Both
    D. Neither

336. Hypercalcemia

337. Cushing's syndrome

338. Hypertension

Questions 339–340:
    A. Cancer antigen 125
    B. Carcinoembryonic antigen (CEA)
    C. Both
    D. Neither

339. Is useful as a screening test for cancer

340. A rise in titer after surgery is indicative of recurrent disease

Explanatory Answers

241. D. Wound infection is the most common complication, occurring in about 30% of cases. (Ref. 20, p. 222)

242. D. Surgical removal alone is capable of curing 80% of stage I disease. (Ref. 20, pp. 160–161)

243. B. A painless mass in the breast is the single most common presenting complaint of patients with underlying breast carcinoma. (Ref. 20, p. 157)

244. A. The reconstruction of the wound is the most important aspect of healing by primary intention. (Ref. 21, p. 6)

245. E. Stainless steel and other wire sutures (silver, tantalum) are not absorbed and are the strongest sutures. (Ref. 21, p. 11)

246. D. When undergoing elective surgery, if there is no indication of coagulopathy, as in a patient who is otherwise healthy, no laboratory tests for bleeding problems are indicated. However, a frozen plasma sample should be kept so that in the rare instance that bleeding diathesis is encountered, an accurate diagnosis can be made. (Ref. 21, p. 31)

247. D. For blood loss up to 20%, administration of lactated Ringer's solution alone may be sufficient. (Ref. 21, p. 43)

248. C. Enlargement of the epitrochlear and axillary nodes should be investigated, since the red streaks indicate local infection of the lymphatic system. (Ref. 21, pp. 48–49)

249. C. The spleen is the most commonly ruptured intraabdominal organ, despite its small size and protection by the left lower rib cage. (Ref. 21, p. 175)

250. B. According to Cope, the goal of the workup is to make the diagnosis utilizing history and physical exam within 15 to 30 minutes so that definitive treatment can be started, and morbidity and mortality rates are decreased. (Ref. 24, p. 5)

251. C. Virchow's triad of stasis, endothelial injury, and hypercoagulability is considered central in the pathogenesis of deep vein thrombosis. (Ref. 21, p. 308)

252. A. Atelectasis is the most likely cause of fever during the first 24 hours postop. The other etiologies usually occur several days after surgery. (Ref. 21, pp. 75–76)

253. C. Approximately 74% of all breast cancers are infiltrating ductal carcinomas. (Ref. 21, p. 140)

254. D. The pain of acute cholecystitis is often referred to the tip of the right scapula. (Ref. 21, p. 158)

255. B. Decompression usually can be performed using a soft rubber rectal tube. Operative procedures would be reserved for cases where the rectal tube was not effective or with recurrence or strangulation. (Ref. 21, p. 238)

256. A. Any abdominal operation is the most common cause of paralytic ileus.(Ref. 21, p. 240)

257. B. Diffuse intestinal dilation is consistent with paralytic ileus. Mechanical bowel obstruction would more likely have localized air–fluid levels. (Ref. 21, p. 240)

258. B. All wounds are weakest approximately 5 to 7 days after injury. (Ref. 19, p. 22)

259. D. Short-term smoking cessation decreases blood levels of carbon monoxide, leaving more hemoglobin available for oxygen transport. The paralyzing effect of smoke on mucociliary transport also may be improved. (Ref. 19, p. 87)

260. D. In such patients, a hematocrit of 25% or hemoglobin of 8 g/dL allows for adequate tissue oxygenation. Patients with longstanding anemia, such as those with chronic renal failure, have increased cardiac output and other compensatory mechanisms, and need not be transfused preoperatively even if the hematocrit drops well below 25%. (Ref. 19, p. 91)

261. B. Protamine is given to reverse rapidly the effects of heparin, while fresh frozen plasma or vitamin K are given to reverse the effects of coumadin. (Ref. 19, p. 91)

262. A. The activated partial thromboplastin time, which measures the activity of the intrinsic coagulation system, is the most sensitive test for establishing the effects of heparin. (Ref. 19, p. 114)

263. A. Many factors interfere with the interpretation of the absolute lymphocyte count, which make its use as a marker for visceral protein malnutrition fairly imprecise and nonspecific. Albumin is the most commonly used analyte for assessing visceral protein stores. Serum transferrin may also be used to assess protein stores and is used to monitor the effects of supplemental albumin on protein stores. Delayed cutaneous hypersensitivity is the most practical test for assessing immunocompetence, which is correlated with visceral protein stores. Midarm muscle circumference is used to assess the somatic or skeletal muscle protein stores. (Ref. 19, p. 134)

264. B. The description is consistent with superficial second-degree burn. (Ref. 19, p. 177)

265. D. For all types of organ donation, the donor must have no intercurrent infection, no previous history of communicable disease, nor intercurrent disease of the organ intended for donation. Compatible weight or body build is not important for kidney or pancreas transplants, but is important for heart, liver, or heart–lung transplants. It is not a universal criteria. (Ref. 19, p. 212)

266. A. The description of the lucid interval, that time after injury when the patient is conscious and apparently free from neurologic problems, is characteristic of epidural hematoma. As the hematoma enlarges, compression of the brain occurs. Coma and death can occur if the hematoma is not evacuated immediately. (Ref. 19, p. 216)

267. E. Physical therapy is added to the therapeutic plan for the management of lumbar disc herniation only after the acute episode is over. The other listed therapies are appropriate during the acute lumbar disc herniation treatment. (Ref. 19, pp. 219–220)

268. A. About 75% of all renal calculi in the United States are composed of two calcium-containing compounds: calcium oxalate and calcium phosphate. Only 15% are from struvite, 8% from uric acid, and 1% from cystine. (Ref. 19, p. 392)

269. E. Ventricular septal defect comprises 25% of the cases of congenital heart disease. The other etiologies account for the percentage of cases as follows: atrial septal defect, 10%; coarctation of the aorta, 5%; tetralogy of Fallot, 10% to 15%; transposition of the great vessels, 10%. (Ref. 19, p. 428)

270. D. Pulmonary embolism is difficult to diagnose due to the fact that the classic signs only occur in about 35% of patients. The classic signs of dyspnea, pleuritic chest pain, apprehension, cough, hemoptysis, and syncope are similar to other cardiorespiratory disorders such as pneumonia, atelectasis, and acute myocardial infarction. Since 11% of patients die within the first hour, it is imperative that rapid diagnosis be made so that definitive treatment may be instituted. (Ref. 19, p. 450)

271. B. The treatment of choice is to resect all aneurysms 5 cm or larger, as determined by imaging, and replace them with interposition grafts. (Ref. 23, p. 402)

272. D. Hereditary spherocytosis, an autosomal dominant trait, is a condition that causes the red blood cells to be spherical, rather than the normal biconcave disk shape. The spleen is almost always enlarged and splenectomy is the treatment of choice in most cases. With acquired hemolytic anemias, removal of the offending agent (drug, chemical, or bacteria), short-term treatment with corticosteroids and transfusion are the treatments of choice. Hereditary elliptocytosis causes only mild hemolysis without anemia or splenomegaly. Splenectomy usually is not indicated. The hereditary anemia associated with G-6-PD deficiency seldom causes splenomegaly, and patients do not benefit from splenectomy. With sickle cell anemia, a few patients may benefit from splenectomy when there is marked splenomegaly early in the course of the disease and when transfusion requirements are high. In most cases, by early adulthood, the spleen is rendered dysfunctional due to multiple splenic infarcts and subsequent atrophy. (Ref. 19, p. 475)

273. A. Infection of the conjunctiva and eyelids is associated with enlargement in the anterior auricular lymph nodes. Dental infection is more likely to be associated with posterior cervical and submental nodes. Oral cavity or pharyngeal infections more likely are associated with anterior cervical nodes. Scalp infection more likely affects posterior cervical, submental, or occipital nodes. Tuberculosis affects nodes in the cervical or submental areas. (Ref. 19, p. 478)

274. E. Pilonidal cysts are usually treated with incision and drainage;

antibiotics are only indicated if the patient is immunosuppressed or has valvular heart disease. (Ref. 19, p. 505)

275. A. Hyperfunctioning (hot) nodules are virtually never malignant. The main objective of the workup of is to detect malignancy. Many etiologies for formation of solitary nodules (benign cysts, thyroiditis, colloid nodule) often may regress with T4 administration. Most thyroid nodules are benign and do not require surgical intervention unless the nodule is very large and it causes mechanical or cosmetic symptoms. (Ref. 19, p. 552)

276. D. Since splenectomized patients have a >50 times risk for overwhelming sepsis from mucopolysaccharide-encapsulated organisms (pneumococci, meningococci, and *H. influenzae)*, and since death occurs in 50% to 80% of patients so afflicted, splenectomy should be avoided when possible in children and undertaken in adults only when it cannot be satisfactorily repaired. (Ref. 21, p. 175)

277. C. Diverticulitis is common in older adults because they frequently have diverticulosis. Appendicitis may rarely be on the left side, but is usually on the right. Pain from colon cancer is usually felt on the right (cecal lesions), and is painless if affecting the left colon. The pain of urinary tract infection is more suprapubic, and would be in parts of the right and left lower quadrants. Sigmoid volvulus is a left lower quadrant problem and is common in the elderly; however, the pain is described as crampy. (Ref. 19, pp. 328–329)

278. A. Benign adnexal masses are more likely to be unilateral. Malignant masses are more likely bilateral, fixed, irregular, solid, and large (>10 cm). (Ref. 19, p. 415)

279. D. Pseudocyst has an incidence of 2% to 3%, and is the most common complication of acute pancreatitis. Although pancreatic cellulitis (phlegmon) and abscess may occur, they are not seen as frequently. Pancreatic fistula is seen only following surgical intervention or trauma. (Ref. 19, pp. 366–367)

280. B. Carotid endarterectomy is considered the treatment of choice because there is a ten-fold decreased risk of stroke after the procedure is performed. The low neurologic morbidity and mortality rates, 1% to 2% and less than 1%, respectively, make the operation an attractive option. (Ref. 19, pp. 222–223)

281. B. Ninety percent of all disc disease affects L4-5 or L5-S1. (Ref. 19, p. 224)

282. C. Although women who have risk factors should begin at an earlier age, all women are considered to be at high risk for breast cancer by age 50 and should begin a schedule of annual mammography at that time. (Ref. 19, p. 526)

283. E. The size of a mass should be documented using only metric measurements. (Ref. 19, p. 6)

284. A. Use of an amebicidal drug like metronidazole is effective in nearly 100% of cases of amebic liver abscess. If a patient fails to respond to drug therapy, then the abscess should be aspirated. (Ref. 19, p. 346)

285. C. Patients with well-controlled seizures on anticonvulsants should continue drugs during the perioperative period. The drug should be switched to a parenteral route during the operative period, until the patient is tolerating oral feedings. These patients may have surgery without being evaluated by a neurologist for clearance. Surgery is not contraindicated in such patients. Clinicians should be vigilant for the conditions of uremia, hyponatremia, and hypernatremia because these conditions may induce seizures. (Ref. 23, p. 74)

286. C. Patients with testicular torsion usually exhibit a tender testicle which lies in the transverse position and is higher in the scrotum than the opposite testicle. The pain is not relieved by scrotal elevation. (Ref. 23, p. 851)

287. D. Fluid resuscitation should be administered as shown in the table below.

Time since burn occurred	Proportion of the calculated fluid volume
First eight hours	½
Second eight hours	¼
Third eight hours	¼

(Ref. 23, p. 126)

288. B. Using the rule of nines, the percent is calculated as follows: anterior arm, 4.5%; anterior leg, 9%. The total burn would be 13.5% of total body surface area. (Ref. 23, p. 124)

289. C. Any underlying cause of the abscess should be treated. Incision and drainage is immediately performed so that tissue is not further destroyed and extension of the infection into the scrotum, thighs, or abdomen is avoided. (Ref. 23, p. 507)

290. A. A palpable thrill that is throughout the cardiac cycle is associated with arteriovenous fistula. The thrill associated with severe stenosis is felt during systole. (Ref. 23, p. 895)

291. B. The positive estrogen receptor assay (ERA) is associated with the effectiveness of hormonal manipulation as the therapy of choice after surgery. These manipulations may include estrogens, antiestrogens, endocrine ablation, or androgens. A negative ERA is associated with the need for chemotherapy. The test does not correlate with the degree of tumor differentiation or the extent of nodal involvement. (Ref. 22, p. 575)

292. D. Measurement of the blood glucose level is the single best test for determining insulin requirements. Levels above 250 mg/dL are undesirable and should be treated with insulin because of the risk associated with fluid depletion from osmotic diuresis. This process compounds the problem of fluid depletion which may be caused by other factors during the immediate postoperative period. (Ref. 23, p. 71)

293. E. Any sign of metastatic disease would confer a worse prognosis. (Ref. 20, pp. 166–167)

294. E. For such patients, all of the treatments should be instituted. (Ref. 21, p. 50)

295. E. All of these are problems associated with inadequate wound drainage. (Ref. 21, p. 11)

296. E. Aspirin, nonsteroidal antiinflammatory drugs (NSAIDS), or high-dose semisynthetic penicillin therapy can affect platelet functioning. Both poor dietary intake and antibiotic therapy are associated with vitamin K deficiency. Binge drinking of alcohol can cause defective platelet functioning at the time of bingeing and thrombocytopenia a few days later. (Ref. 21, p. 31)

297. A. It would be appropriate to give penicillin, to apply warm soaks and to elevate the leg. The extremity should be immobilized, if possible—not excessively moved, as with range of motion exercises. (Ref. 21, p. 48)

298. C. Alcohol intake and gallstones make up the majority of cases of acute pancreatitis. Trauma may cause acute pancreatitis, but is not as common a cause. (Ref. 21, p. 165)

299. A. According to Cope, the pain, usually umbilical or epigastric, precedes the vomiting which, in turn, precedes fever. The diagnosis of appendicitis should be in doubt if these symptoms do not occur in order. Testicular pain is an uncommon symptom of appendicitis. (Ref. 24, pp. 69–76)

300. C. The direct hernia is identified by its anatomical location, which is medial to the inferior deep epigastric artery. The etiology is most likely from wear and tear. The hernia need not be surgically repaired unless the patient is symptomatic, since direct hernias rarely incarcerate or strangulate due to the large size neck of the hernia sac. Direct hernias are the second most common type of hernia. (Ref. 21, p. 190)

301. C. Surgery may be necessary for patients whose hernias become large in size or have ulceration, bleeding, or stenosis as complications. (Ref. 21, p. 194)

302. A. Surgery is definitely indicated for bleeding, obstruction, and perforation. Although surgery may be performed for recurrent ulcers, some respond to cimetidine or ranitidine. (Ref. 21, p. 198)

303. E. All of the tests listed are helpful in determining the risk for morbidity and mortality due to malnutrition in surgical patients. (Ref. 21, p. 58)

304. A. Risks include those in choices 1, 2, and 3, and also rhythm other than sinus or premature atrial contractions on preoperative EKG; more than five premature ventricular contractions per minute at any time before the operation; an intraperitoneal, intrathoracic or aortic operation; important valvular stenosis; an emergency operation; and poor general condition. (Ref. 21, p. 64)

305. A. Adhesion and hernias comprise about 70% of all obstructions in adults. Tumors cause about 15% of all bowel obstructions, but nearly all of large bowel obstructions. Intussception is rare in adults. (Ref. 21, p. 237)

306. C. Fecal impaction and gallstone ileus are the most common causes of obturation in more advanced countries. Parasitic infections are more common in underdeveloped areas and bezoars are found in mentally defective patients. (Ref. 21, p. 239)

307. E. All of the symptoms, in any combination, are associated with uncomplicated hemorrhoids. (Ref. 21, p. 246)

308. E. All of the listed factors, along with malnutrition, are considered to be risk factors for postoperative pneumonia. (Ref. 19, p. 22)

309. A. As part of initial coma resuscitation, dextrose can be given to reverse the coma associated with hypoglycemia. Narcan can reverse the effects of an overdose of narcotics, which would be another common cause of coma. Thiamine is given to protect the alcoholic patient from developing Wernicke's syndrome from the administration of glucose. Antibiotics would not have any immediate effect on the patient's coma status, so they would not be given at this time. Antibiotics may be given later, if indicated. (Ref. 19, p. 39)

310. B. Since epinephrine acts to constrict arteries, its use is contraindicated in body areas which have limited blood supply for normal anatomic reasons. Also, its use would be limited in patients with reduced blood supplies due to pathologic changes. Epinephrine should not be used in contaminated wounds because local vasoconstriction may decrease local infection defense mechanisms. The total quantity injected should not exceed 1 mg. (Ref. 19, p. 46)

311. A. Elective operations during the first trimester of pregnancy should be avoided due to the concern about the effects of surgery and anesthesia on the developing fetus during its time of organogenesis. After 12 weeks gestation, all pregnant patients are considered to have a "full stomach" because of decreased gastric emptying. Therefore, rapid induction anesthesia would be warranted for surgery requiring general anesthesia. Due to the large uterus exerting pressure on the vena cava, supine hypotension syndrome may occur during the last trimester when the patient is in the supine position. The fetus should be monitored by constant Doppler monitoring during surgery. (Ref. 19, p. 89)

312. C. Positive pleural effusion cytology and Horner's syndrome indicate widespread involvement not amenable to resection. Tumors located in the periphery or those without extension past the hilum are more likely to be able to be resected. (Ref. 19, p. 275)

313. B. Patients with intractable pain who fail to respond to medical therapy and those with gastric outlet obstruction should have definitive ulcer surgery. For acute perforation, after closure of the perforation with an omental patch, definitive ulcer surgery would be performed only on otherwise healthy individuals with a history suggestive of chronic disease. Acute hemorrhage may be arrested in about 65% of patients with conservative medical therapy. Definitive ulcer surgery would be indicated, however, with patients who had continued, massive, or recurrent bleeding. (Ref. 19, p. 291)

314. D. In order to be stage IV, the tumor must have distant metastases, so the only tumor with distant metastases would be $T_1 N_1 M_1$. (Ref. 19, p. 532)

315. B. The most common evidence of injury to the kidneys, ureters, or bladder is gross or microscopic hematuria. The amount of hematuria does not correlate well with the extent of injury. (Ref. 19, p. 394)

316. B. Testicular carcinomas are found most frequently in young men, ages 20 to 40, and present with painless enlargement. The most common cell patterns are single cell (60% of all testicular tumors) with seminoma (35%), embryonal cell (20%), teratocarcinoma (5%), and choriocarcinoma (<1%). Mixed cell tumors comprise the other 40%. Overall survival rates are good with appropriate surgery, radiotherapy, and chemotherapy, depending on the tumor type, even for patients with metastatic disease. (Ref. 19, pp. 396–397)

317. A. Varicosities are mostly a cosmetic problem, but need to be differentiated from those caused by pelvic tumors, venous obstruction within the abdomen, or cardiac failure. The varicosities are related to venous valvular incompetence. Varicosities can be treated successfully with the three measures mentioned. There is little risk for development of large pulmonary emboli because the varicosities are superficial—not deep. (Ref. 19, pp. 445–447)

318. B. The pain of intermittent claudication may be in the thigh, buttocks, or, most likely, in the calf, and is experienced upon walking. The pain subsides with rest. Impotence may be experienced by the patient due to decreased blood flow and is termed Leriche's syndrome. Vascular disease in the extremities suggests vascular disease elsewhere, so the workup should include tests to determine the competency of the entire vascular system. (Ref. 19, p. 463)

319. E. Bilateral inferior laryngeal nerve injury usually requires endotracheal intubation and/or tracheostomy for airway control. Unilateral nerve injury results in various degrees of hoarseness, but may be asymptomatic. Injury to the superior laryngeal nerves results in loss of sensation to the larynx and pyriform sinus, with an increased chance of aspiration resulting. Voice quality and strength may also change. The clinical manifestations of hypoparathyroidism may be transient (due to edema) or permanent (due to removal of the parathyroid glands or their infarction, due to decreased blood supply). Wound hemorrhage is possible. A small amount of blood in the wound space can cause compression of the airway. (Ref. 19, p. 555)

320. E. Since many of the diseases of lymph nodes are related to cancer or infection, all of the tests may be appropriate. (Ref. 19, p. 478)

321. C. Myxomas are found in the left atrium about 75% of the time. Patients do exhibit symptoms of systemic embolization and do have a positional heart murmur. Resection is the treatment of choice, and morbidity and mortality are usually low. (Ref. 19, pp. 442–443)

322. A. Atherosclerosis is seen in the saphenous vein grafts which have been in place for many years. Reduced rates are seen with internal mammary vein grafts. (Ref. 23, p. 1123)

323. E. All are complications of endoscopic spincterotomy. (Ref. 23, p. 567)

324. A. An increased amount of conversation in the operating room has been associated with increased rates of postoperative wound infection; therefore, limiting unnecessary conversation would be prudent. It has been demonstrated that a five-minute initial scrub of hands of operative personnel yields the same results as a ten-minute initial scrub. Paper drapes are preferable to cloth drapes, because paper drapes are impervious to bacteria and transmission of bacteria is decreased. Cloth drapes are prone to contamination from the patient's skin flora, especially when the cloth drape gets wet. Shaving of the operative site is a method that is being reassessed. Studies have shown that patients have lower rates of postoperative wound infection when the hair is removed by use of a depilatory or when the hair is left in place. (Ref. 23, p. 133)

325. A. Routine preoperative chest films yield little information in healthy patients, but are valuable for patients with known or suspected pulmonary disease. (Ref. 19, p. 88)

326. A.   In a direct hernia, the hernia sac arises in Hesselbach's triangle,
327. B.   medial to the inferior deep epigastric artery, and just above the
328. D.   pubic tubercle. Indirect hernias protrude through the inguinal ring along the course of the inguinal canal. These hernias often descend into the scrotum and arise lateral to the deep inferior epigastric artery. Both direct and indirect inguinal hernias are more common in men. Femoral hernias are more common in women. (Ref. 21, p. 190)

329. A.   Adenocarcinomas are usually more peripheral in location.
330. A.   Large cell carcinomas are peripheral lesions often greater than
331. B.   4 cm. Small cell tumors usually appear as hilar abnormalities. (Ref. 19, p. 257)

332. A.   Patients with ulcerative colitis are more at risk for toxic
333. C.   megacolon. Bloody diarrhea can be seen with both ulcerative
334. A.   colitis and granulomatous colitis; however, the bleeding is usu-
335. B.   ally more prevalent with ulcerative colitis. There is an increased risk for colon cancer in patients who have had ulcerative colitis for ten years or more. The "skip" pattern is typical for granulomatous colitis, since some segments of the bowel are free from disease. (Ref. 19, pp. 320–322)

336. D.   Parathyroid tumors and Hodgkin's disease are related to the
337. B.   development of hypercalcemia. Cushing's syndrome is related
338. A.   to ectopic ACTH secretion of carcinoid. Hypertension is related to catecholamine secreting pheochromocytomas. (Ref. 23, p. 1025)

339. D.   Neither test is considered adequate as a screening test for can-
340. C.   cer, due to numerous conditions that increase both antigens. For both, a rise in the titer from the preoperative level is indicative of recurrent disease. Cancer antigen 125 is used to follow patients with ovarian cancer, while carcinoembryonic antigen is used to follow patients with colon tumors. (Ref. 22, pp. 577, 589)

8 Pediatrics

DIRECTIONS (Questions 341–410): Each of the questions or incomplete statements below is followed by four or five suggested answers or completions. Select the **one** that is best in each case.

341. All of the following vaccinations contain live viruses **EXCEPT**
- **A.** tetanus
- **B.** polio
- **C.** measles
- **D.** mumps

342. The following are all adverse effects of vaccination for pertussis (whooping cough) **EXCEPT**
- **A.** convulsions
- **B.** diarrhea
- **C.** syncopal episode
- **D.** inconsolable crying for longer than three hours

343. Contraindications for vaccination include all of the following **EXCEPT**
- **A.** employment in a day-care setting
- **B.** fever
- **C.** progressive neurological disorder
- **D.** history of seizures

344. The *H. influenzae* vaccination is given to protect against all of the following **EXCEPT**
A. otitis media
B. meningitis
C. pneumonia
D. osteomyelitis

345. A four-month-old infant presents to the emergency room with retractions and tachypnea. Her mother says that the child has been ill for several days, but is now sicker. The child has no fever and exam reveals coarse inspiratory and expiratory breath sounds throughout the chest. The chest x-ray reveals low diaphragms and areas of linear atelectasis. There is no previous history of similar episodes. What is a likely diagnosis?
A. Asthma
B. Congestive heart failure
C. Bronchiolitis
D. Pneumonia

346. Symptoms associated with meningitis in newborns include all of the following **EXCEPT**
A. temperature instability
B. severe headache
C. bulging or full fontanelle
D. jaundice

347. Which of the following organisms is the **MOST** common cause of meningitis in children?
A. *S. pneumoniae*
B. *H. influenzae*
C. *Neisseria meningitidis*
D. *Staphylococcus aureus*

348. All of the following are appropriate for treatment of meningitis caused by *H. influenzae* in children greater than one month of age **EXCEPT**
A. third-generation cephalosporins
B. aminoglycosides
C. tetracycline
D. chloramphenicol

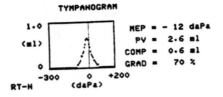

Type A Normal

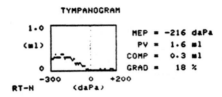

Type C Retracted

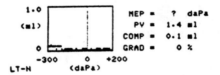

Type B Flat

Figure 2

349. Which of the tympanograms in Figure 2 would demonstrate both air and fluid behind the ear drum?
   A. Normal
   B. Retracted
   C. Flat
   D. Inverted

350. Antibiotics appropriate for an initial or uncomplicated otitis media include all of the following **EXCEPT**
   A. pediazole
   B. amoxicillin
   C. both A and B
   D. erythromycin

351. All of the following contribute to anemia in infants fed only cow's milk **EXCEPT**
   A. inadequate amounts of iron in cow's milk
   B. occult bleeding of the GI tract
   C. supplementary feeds introduced early in the first year of life may decrease absorption of iron
   D. the mother of the infant may give less cow's milk because it is more expensive

352. The leading cause of accidents in children who ride in the back of family trucks is
   A. major head trauma
   B. minor head trauma
   C. fractures
   D. abrasions

353. Common prenatal conditions associated with small-for-gestational-age newborns include all of the following **EXCEPT**
   A. maternal diabetes
   B. placental insufficiency
   C. toxemia of pregnancy
   D. intrauterine infections

354. Which of the following conditions does **NOT** occur in small-for-gestational-age infants?
   A. Hypoglycemia
   B. Hypothermia
   C. Sepsis
   D. Fracture of the clavicle

355. Which of the following should be provided to a breast-fed infant?
   A. Calcium
   B. Iron
   C. Vitamin E
   D. Vitamin D

356. Cardiac lesions are frequently associated with
   A. failure to thrive
   B. short stature
   C. both choice A and choice B
   D. neither choice A nor choice B

357. Blood from the placenta reenters the fetal circulation via the
   A. patent ductus arteriosus
   B. ductus venosus
   C. ductus communis
   D. ductus efferent

358. Each of the following statements is true about failure to thrive (FTT) **EXCEPT**
   A. the first growth parameter to be affected is the head circumference
   B. hospitalization is not often necessary to discover the etiology of FTT
   C. an organic cause for FTT would be malabsorption of calories
   D. factors associated with FTT may include young parents, economic stress, or single parenthood

359. The most obvious findings in a child who is failing to thrive include all of the following **EXCEPT**
   A. mental retardation
   B. lack of weight gain
   C. delayed gross motor activity
   D. withdrawal from social interaction

360. All of the following statements about sinusitis in children are true **EXCEPT**
   A. persistent cough may be the only symptom
   B. teeth may be tender in maxillary sinusitis
   C. ampicillin or amoxicillin are drugs of first choice
   D. a stain may reveal eosinophils

361. All of the following findings on sinus films would be indicative of infection **EXCEPT**
   A. thickened mucosa
   B. air–fluid levels
   C. opacification of the sinus
   D. interstitial markings

362. An eight-year-old girl presents to the emergency room with the abrupt onset of shaking chills, fever, and a productive cough. She is tachycardic, tachypneic, and has rales audible in her right mid-lung field. The chest x-ray reveals an infiltrate in her right mid-lung field. Which is the **MOST** likely diagnosis and treatment?
   A. Pneumococcal pneumonia/penicillin
   B. Mycoplasma pneumonia/penicillin
   C. Pneumococcal pneumonia/erythromycin
   D. Mycoplasma pneumonia/erythromycin

363. Which of the following are appropriate areas of inquiry for an adolescent interview?
   A. School
   B. Extracurricular activities
   C. Drug and alcohol use
   D. Peer relationships
   E. All of the above

364. While on rounds at the newborn nursery, you are called to see a 12-hour-old infant who has begun convulsing. The **FIRST** method of treatment would be
   A. IV Valium
   B. Calcium gluconate
   C. IV vitamin B_6
   D. IV glucose

365. Contraindications to induction of emesis in childhood poisoning include all of the following **EXCEPT**
   A. ingestion of turpentine
   B. rapidly increasing drowsiness
   C. ingestion of drain cleaner
   D. ingestion of iron preparations

366. Local side-effects of topical corticosteroids may include all of the following **EXCEPT**
  A. atrophy
  B. secondary infections, such as yeast
  C. hypopigmentation
  D. jaundice

367. While performing an initial physical on a newborn infant, you notice simian creases, epicanthal folds, and a heart murmur. A preliminary diagnosis would be
  A. Down's syndrome
  B. tetralogy of Fallot
  C. Turner's syndrome
  D. fetal rubella syndrome

368. Factors common in children with asthma may include all of the following **EXCEPT**
  A. multifactorial heredity
  B. prior to puberty, it is more common in girls
  C. many children may "outgrow" their asthma because their airways become larger in diameter
  D. strong family history for asthma is common

369. Pathophysiology associated with asthma may include all of the following **EXCEPT**
  A. collapse of the airway
  B. spasm of smooth muscle
  C. intraluminal collection of mucus
  D. edema of mucous membranes

370. A 15-year-old with asthma calls to find out her theophylline level. You tell her that it is 10 μ/dL, which is normal. She is presently taking theophylline capsules and wants to continue them. Each capsule may contain 100, 200, or 300 mg. She weighs 60 kg. Which of the following regimens would be appropriate for her?
  A. 300 mg po q 6 hr
  B. 200 mg po q 6 hr
  C. 100 mg po q 6 hr
  D. 600 mg po q 6 hr

371. Asthma in children is usually associated with all of the following **EXCEPT**
A. allergic rhinitis
B. atopic dermatitis
C. nasal polyps
D. eosinophilia

372. Cystic fibrosis may include all of the following **EXCEPT**
A. chronic cough
B. failure to thrive
C. constipation
D. fatty stools

373. All of the following statements about fungal infections of the scalp are true **EXCEPT**
A. sporicidal shampoos will kill spores after use for about two weeks
B. budding hyphae can be seen on KOH prep when scrapings are examined
C. they can be treated with topical antifungal agents
D. they may require antibiotics if the skin becomes secondarily infected with bacteria

374. An eight-year-old girl is brought to the clinic because her parents noticed several vesicular lesions on her trunk. The child brought them to the attention of her parents by asking for something for itching. She had not been feeling well for a couple of days prior to that, and had had fever, headaches, and malaise. A likely diagnosis is
A. rubella
B. chicken pox
C. scarlet fever
D. measles

375. The following statements about TB skin testing are true **EXCEPT**
A. the most reliable test is the Mantoux test
B. use of a TB skin test in someone with active disease may result in a negative reaction
C. a positive TB skin is greater than 15 mm in diameter
D. the initial TB skin test should be given when a child is 12 to 15 months of age

376. The highest rate of tuberculosis in children in the United States is among which group?
A. American Indians/Eskimos
B. Hispanics
C. Blacks
D. Asians

377. All of the following are frequent signs and symptoms of tuberculosis in children **EXCEPT**
A. trunchal obesity
B. night sweats
C. failure to thrive
D. persistent cough

378. An innocent murmur of school-age children characterized by a low-pitched systolic murmur that is best heard between the apex and the lower left sternal border is called
A. Still's murmur
B. functional murmur
C. tetralogy of Fallot
D. supraventricular arterial bruit

379. With the infant supine and the neck turned to one side, the infant will extend the arm and leg on the same side and will flex the arm and leg on the opposite side. Which of the following terms describes this reflex in infants?
A. Moro reflex
B. Babinski reflex
C. Tonic neck reflex
D. Ankle clonus

380. A seizure that includes loss of consciousness, staring, or eye fluttering, but no other motor involvement, is termed
A. partial complex seizure
B. absence (petit mal) seizure
C. tonic-clonic seizure
D. partial simple seizure

381. Which of the following medications is recommended for the seizure disorder identified in question 380?
- **A.** Phenytoin (Dilantin)
- **B.** Phenobarbital
- **C.** Valproic acid (Depakote)
- **D.** Diazepam (Valium)

382. All of the following laboratory evaluations are appropriate to evaluate a patient who receives the medication recommended in question 381 **EXCEPT**
- **A.** complete blood count, including platelets
- **B.** liver function studies
- **C.** valproic acid level
- **D.** cardiac enzymes

383. All of the following conditions discovered during the evaluation of a child with headaches would warrant a CT scan **EXCEPT**
- **A.** a neurologic abnormality
- **B.** a child three years or less in age
- **C.** a child with short stature or failure to thrive
- **D.** a normal ophthalmologic examination

384. Which of the following conditions should be suspected in a newborn who does not pass meconium by 24 hours of age, is not eating well, has a distended abdomen, and is vomiting?
- **A.** Pyloric stenosis
- **B.** Hirschsprung's disease
- **C.** Constipation
- **D.** Anal fissure

385. All of the following statements about congenital syphilis are true **EXCEPT**
- **A.** the disease is usually spread during the birth process
- **B.** the rash may be vesicular, bullous, maculopapular, or resemble erythema multiforme
- **C.** other symptoms may include jaundice, pneumonia, or hepatosplenomegaly
- **D.** diagnosis includes a VDRL and FTA on CNS fluid

386. An 18-month-old child accompanied his parents on a visit to Acapulco, Mexico. While there, the child began to have diarrhea and diminished appetite. His parents had had some nausea and diarrhea, also, but had recovered at the time of the child's visit. The child was brought to the doctor because of the onset of bloody diarrhea. Which of the following is/are appropriate for initial evaluation?
   A. Stain of stool for white blood cells and microorganisms
   B. Stool for ova and parasites
   C. Stool for culture and sensitivity
   D. Duodenal aspirate for giardia
   E. All of the above

387. All of the following factors contribute to physiologic jaundice **EXCEPT**
   A. delay in passage of meconium
   B. destruction of fetal hemoglobin
   C. deficient glucuronyltransferase in the liver
   D. Rh^+ baby as the offspring of Rh^- mother

388. Which of the following clinical findings is/are associated with necrotizing enterocolitis?
   A. Abdominal distention
   B. Bloody stools
   C. Air in the bowel wall on plain radiographs
   D. All of the above

389. A four-year-old male is brought in for medical attention after a two-month history of fatigue, intermittent fever to unknown degree, and spots on his abdomen. Your exam reveals a listless child who appears pale. He tells you that his joints have ached and motions over his thighs and shins to indicate where he has discomfort. No elevation in his temperature is noted at the time of his exam. You do discover petechiae on his palate, some bruising on his trunk, a liver that is enlarged, as well as a palpable spleen. An appropriate initial laboratory evaluation includes which of the following?
   A. Complete blood count
   B. C-reactive protein
   C. Blood cultures
   D. Radiographs of involved limbs
   E. All of the above

390. The CBC report reveals a hemoglobin of 8 with a hematocrit of 24.1, a white blood cell count of 3000, and thrombocytopenia. All of the other reports reveal normal findings and negative blood cultures. You suspect that the child may have which of the following?
A. Leukemia
B. Brain tumor
C. Juvenile rheumatoid arthritis
D. Systemic lupus erythematosus

391. All of the following statements about cryptorchidism are true **EX-CEPT**
A. it is defined as the failure of the testes to be present at the bottom of the scrotal sac at the time of birth
B. this condition is not associated with a decreased number of spermatogonia in the undescended testis
C. many times, the undescended testis can be brought into an anatomically normal position by the administration of HCG
D. the undescended testis has a higher rate of testicular tumors

392. Causes of gynecomastia may include all of the following **EXCEPT**
A. puberty
B. ingestion of certain drugs (eg, cimetidine or estrogens)
C. Klinefelter's syndrome
D. lack of exercise as a prepubertal child

393. All of the following statements about enuresis are true **EXCEPT**
A. this condition is much more common in girls
B. children are usually three years of age before they can control bladder function most of the time
C. children with enuresis have a lower mean bone age, later sexual maturation, and lower average height compared to children who do not have this condition
D. children with enuresis have a reduced functional bladder capacity

394. Treatment for enuresis (after an organic cause is excluded) includes all of the following **EXCEPT**
   A. education of the child as to how common this condition is so as to allay anxiety and embarrassment that he or she feels about it
   B. behavior modification, including a reward system for a dry bed as well as responsibility for changing a wet bed
   C. scolding the child because he appears lazy and won't stay dry
   D. bladder training exercises during the day to help improve functional bladder capacity

395. Which of the following must be considered in the differential diagnosis for a child undergoing evaluation for encopresis?
   A. Hirschsprung's disease
   B. Chronic cocaine or phenothiazine use
   C. Anal or rectal stenosis
   D. Sensory or motor defects of the anorectum or muscles of the pelvic floor
   E. All of the above

396. Which of the following **CORRECTLY** identifies a patient with anorexia nervosa?
   A. Intense fear of being overweight, with onset prior to age 25
   B. Weight loss of at least 25% of original body weight
   C. Maintaining body weight at the minimum of normal for height
   D. Amenorrhea

397. All of the following can cause a maculopapular rash that is not IgE mediated after the administration of ampicillin **EXCEPT**
   A. infectious mononucleosis
   B. hyperuricemia
   C. administration of allopurinol
   D. choices A and C
   E. all of the above

398. A ten-year-old female is brought for medical attention after the onset of sharp, stabbing chest pains while she attempted to sit up. She describes the pain as "bad" and points to an area on her chest at the left midclavicular portion of her fifth rib. She was resting at the time of her pain, and denies any recent changes in activity, trauma, coughing, or respiratory infection. Physical exam reveals an entirely normal cardiac exam, no pain upon compression of her rib cage, adventitious breath sounds, or pleural rub. Armed with this information, the **MOST** likely diagnosis is

    A. costochondritis
    B. precordial catch syndrome
    C. *Mycoplasma pneumoniae*
    D. esophageal reflux

399. Which of the following terms describes this finding in infants? A raised red, firm, well-circumscribed, partially compressible lesion, found most commonly on the face, scalp, and thorax.

    A. Chemangioma
    B. Spider nevus
    C. Capillary hemangioma
    D. Café-au-lait spots

400. All of the following statements about spina bifida are true **EXCEPT**

    A. meningomyelocoele refers to the exposure of the meninges, spinal cord, and spinal roots
    B. spina bifida is often associated with dermal sinuses, dimples, and lipomas
    C. the lesion is usually located in the thoracic spine
    D. this disorder can be detected prenatally by measuring alpha-fetoprotein in either maternal blood or amniotic fluid

401. All of the following are risk factors for hearing loss in infants **EXCEPT**

    A. birth weight of 1500 grams or less
    B. placenta previa associated with child's prenatal course
    C. seizures
    D. hyperbilirubinemia of greater than 20 mg/100 mL

402. A four-year-old is brought to your clinic with a one-day history of watery discharge and red irritated eyes. She also has a sore throat and fever. She has no previous history of similar episodes. Your examination reveals her pupil, cornea, and vision to be normal. What is the **MOST** likely cause of this condition?
A. Allergic conjunctivitis
B. Viral conjunctivitis
C. Bacterial conjunctivitis
D. Herpetic conjunctivitis

403. The **MOST** common cause of ophthalmia neonatorum is
A. *N. gonorrhoeae*
B. *Chlamydia*
C. herpes simplex
D. *S. aureus*

404. All of the following infections in the newborn period may be caused by *Chlamydia* **EXCEPT**
A. pneumonia
B. otitis media
C. rhinitis
D. urinary tract infection

405. All of the following are clinical signs of congenital dislocation of the hip **EXCEPT**
A. hip click or thump with manipulation of the hip joint
B. inability of the infant to bring himself to a standing position
C. laxity of the hamstrings
D. limping after the infant begins walking

406. An infant who has tenting of his skin, dry mucous membranes, irritability, decreased tearing, and diminished urine output is said to be dehydrated by what percentage?
A. 1%
B. 5% to 10%
C. 10% to 15%
D. Greater than 15%

407. Which of the following intravenous fluids would be appropriate to begin for the child in question 406 even before any laboratory reports have been obtained?
   A. D5W
   B. D5 normal saline
   C. D10W
   D. Ringer's lactate

408. Which of the following are appropriate as prophylaxis for Hepatitis B in the newborn?
   A. Hepatitis B immunoglobin
   B. Hepatitis B vaccine within 12 hours of birth
   C. Hepatitis B booster at 1 and 6 months of age
   D. Choices A and B
   E. All of the above

409. All of the following statements about bacteremia in children are true **EXCEPT**
   A. this condition is most common in children 3 to 24 months of age
   B. the most common etiology is *E. coli*
   C. children with congenital or functional asplenia are at increased risk for bacteremia
   D. a newborn between birth and two months of age who appears septic should have a complete evaluation for sepsis and hospitalization to receive parenteral antibiotics

410. Children who are cared for in day-care centers, as well as their caregivers, are at risk for all of the following infections **EXCEPT**
   A. hepatitis A
   B. rotavirus
   C. giardia
   D. hepatitis B

DIRECTIONS (Questions 411–415): The group of questions below consists of lettered headings followed by a list of numbered words, phrases, or statements. For each numbered word, phrase, or statement, select the **one** lettered heading that is most closely associated with it. Each lettered heading may be selected once, more than once, or not at all.

A. Atopic dermatitis
B. Acne
C. Seborrhea
D. Erythema multiforme
E. Pityriasis rosea

411. Hypersensitivity to a drug, usually sulfa

412. Herald patch

413. Scaly skin, many times associated with itching

414. Pustules, comedos, cysts

415. Oily, scaly skin over face and scalp

Explanatory Answers

341. A. All of the above except tetanus contains live viruses. This is important because those people who have an immunocompromised condition (those receiving chemotherapy; those on steroids; those who have AIDS) and pregnant women should not receive live vaccinations. It is also important to remember that children who receive live viruses will be shedding the virus for several weeks while building immunity. It is equally important to inquire as to whether there is anyone in the child's household who should not be exposed to live viruses. Polio, for instance, is shed from the GI tract up to six weeks after the immunization. (Ref. 33, p. 10)

342. B. Other adverse effects of the vaccine include temperature greater than 105 °F (40.6 °C), encephalitis, somnolence, and thrombocytopenic purpura. If any of the reactions occur, no other pertussis vaccines should be given. It is also not appropriate to give a smaller dose. (Refs. 29, p. 140; 33, p. 10)

343. A. All of the others are contraindications for immunization. Children with seizure disorders must be evaluated on an individual basis to determine whether a vaccine should be given. Other reasons not to administer a vaccine include pregnancy, or being within three months of pregnancy, and immunosuppression. (Ref. 33, p. 10)

344. A. All of the above infections caused by *H. influenzae* can be prevented by this immunization except for the strains that cause otitis. Conjugated forms have now been approved for use in children as young as two months of age. (Refs. 25, p. 21; 33, p. 16)

345. C. This is a classical description of bronchiolitis which is caused by the respiratory syncytical virus. The following supports the diagnosis: there is evidence of lower airway obstruction (low diaphragms, tachypnea), the child is an infant, and there are no similar episodes. Air exchange does not improve after administration of a bronchodilator, whereas it does with asthma. (Ref. 33, pp. 86–89)

346. B. All of the others are signs of meningitis in newborns. Others include color changes, seizures, poor feeding, lethargy, tachypnea, apnea, an abnormal Moro reflex, opisthotonos, and possibly coma. (Ref. 25, p. 1020)

347. B. *H. influenzae* is the most common cause of meningitis in children. Choices A and C are less common causes. (Refs. 25, p. 1022; 30, p. 662)

348. C. Ampicillin and chloramphenicol are the traditional treatment for this type of infection. Third-generation cephalosporins are modifying these choices for treatment with less risk to the patient. Chloramphenicol is toxic to the bone marrow and may cause neutropenia or aplastic anemia. In newborns, this antibiotic may cause the gray baby syndrome. Aminoglycosides cause ototoxicity and renal compromise. Children with meningitis should have their hearing tested. (Refs. 25, p. 1022; 30, pp. 663–664)

349. B. A retracted tympanogram demonstrates negative pressures of less than –100 mm air pressure and greater than 0.3 mL compliance. There is both air and fluid present behind the tympanum. A flat tympanogram has no distinct peak and compliance of less than 0.3 mL. This type is usually associated with middle-ear effusion. A normal tympanogram has a peak compliance at or greater than –100 mm pressure and normal amplitude (see Figure 2). (Ref. 29, pp. 302–303)

350. D. Pediazole and amoxicillin can provide coverage for the two most common organisms that cause otitis media, *S. pneumoniae* and *H. influenzae*, but amoxicillin does not provide quite as broad a spectrum. Pediazole provides coverage to *S. pneumoniae*, but also works against both beta-lactamase producing and non-beta-lactamase producing strains of *H. influenzae*. Another organism, *Branhamella catarrhalis*, is the third most common organism and pediazole works for both beta-lactamase producing and non-beta-lactamase producing strains of this organism, also. Erythromycin is not effective against *H. influenzae*. (Ref. 27, pp. 133–135)

351. D. Usually mothers change the infant's formula to cow's milk because it is less expensive or they are unaware that their infants require supplements for the entire first year of life. Because anemia is so common and infants grow so rapidly in the first year of life, all children should have a screening hemoglobin and hematocrit between 9 and 13 months of age. (Ref. 31, p. 35)

352. B. Motor vehicle accidents are the most common cause of accidents to children. A recent study reported that the most common injury was minor head trauma, which includes loss of consciousness, postconcussive syndrome, and cuts and abrasions. Major head trauma included skull fractures, intracranial bleeds, seizures, and scalp lacerations. (Ref. 35)

353. A. Maternal diabetes results in large-for-gestational-age infants, whereas the other three all result in small-for-gestational-age babies. Small-for-gestational-age babies are those that fall below the tenth percentile in weight for their gestational age. (Ref. 36)

354. D. All of the other conditions may occur in SGA infants. The most common one is hypoglycemia. Factors that contribute to this include fetal malnutrition, hypothermia, respiratory distress syndrome, cerebral damage, and infant of prediabetic (gestational) or diabetic mother. (Ref. 36, pp. 454–455)

355. D. Breast milk may not contain enough vitamin D, especially if the mother is not exposed to sunlight or does not drink fortified cow's milk. (Ref. 29, p. 114)

356. C. (Refs. 29, p. 474; 37, p. 360)

357. A. While the fetus remains in utero, blood reentering fetal circulation is not a problem because blood is funneled through the ductus to the aorta and placenta. It is only when the infant begins to breathe that problems may arise. The pulmonary artery has a lower pressure than does the aorta, and when the ductus remains open, blood will then enter the lower-pressure artery, the pulmonary artery, and go on to the lungs, to cause pulmonary edema. (Ref. 26, p. 987)

358. A. The first growth parameter to be affected is weight, then height, and, finally, head circumference. (Ref. 37, p. 359)

359. A. All of the other findings may be easily assessed during the evaluation; but, in a study by Glazer, one-half of children with FTT also had cognitive function below normal. (Ref. 37, p. 366)

360. D. A smear may reveal segmented neutrophils as a sign of infection, whereas eosinophils are associated with allergies. It is also possible for both conditions to be present at the same time. The symptoms listed, as well as headache, nasal discharge for longer than ten days, or fever, may indicate a sinus infection. Many parents may notice halitosis. (Ref. 30, p. 384)

361. D. The first three findings may all indicate sinusitis, although air–fluid levels are uncommon in children under five years of age. Measurements of mucosal linings greater than 5 mm in adults and 4 mm in children indicates that an infection is likely. (Ref. 30, p. 385)

362. A. This is a classical description of pneumococcal pneumonia and penicillin and cephalosporins are commonly used, although erythromycin can be used for this type of pneumonia, also. (Ref. 30, pp. 683–684)

363. E. All of the concerns listed are appropriate to discuss with an adolescent, as well as sexual activity and relationships with family. These subjects should be discussed in an atmosphere that encourages the adolescent to be open about concerns, without feeling that parents will be told what transpired during the interview unless information is discovered that represents a serious threat to the teenager (eg, plans for suicide). (Ref. 30, p. 43)

354. D. Hypoglycemia is a common cause of neonatal seizures. Treating this condition quickly may alleviate sequelae. (Ref. 29, p. 457)

365. D. Prevention of absorption of iron can be accomplished by inducing vomiting with syrup of ipecac; but, if the child is obtunded, gastric lavage with an NG tube should be used to prevent aspiration. Hydrocarbons cause most of their damage by aspiration into the lungs; lye may reinjure the esophagus if vomiting is induced. (Ref. 30, pp. 715, 724, 721)

366. D. All of the choices except jaundice are side-effects of steroids. Care must also be taken because children are more susceptible "to topical corticosteroid-induced HPA axis suppression because of a larger skin surface area to bodyweight ratio." (Refs. 30, p. 261; 38)

367. A. The description is most consistent with Down's syndrome or Trisomy 21. (Ref. 29, p. 250)

368. B. It is more common in boys prior to puberty. (Ref. 26, p. 495)

369. A. (Ref. 28, p. 155)

370. A. Theophylline is prescribed at 5 mg/kg/dose every six hours. (Ref. 39, p. 27)

371. C. Asthma in children is usually extrinsic or IgE mediated, and all but nasal polyps are associated with this type of asthma. Some children may have a mixed form that includes signs of intrinsic asthma; one of these signs is nasal polyps. (Ref. 28, p. 155)

372. C. Cystic fibrosis is a genetic disorder that includes all of the choices listed except constipation. It is most commonly a disease of the lung and the exocrine portion of the pancreas. (Ref. 26, pp. 926–927)

373. C. Tinea capitis requires systemic griseofulvin because the spores and hyphae invade the hair shaft. It must be given for 6 to 8 weeks to kill all the spores. The shampoos will help kill spores, also. The use of a Wood's lamp has been used, but not all dermatophytes fluoresce when examined. A KOH prep and culture are now recommended for diagnosis. (Ref. 30, pp. 289–291)

374. B. Chicken pox is characterized by a vesicular rash that starts as a macular rash, which then becomes vesicular, then ruptures, and finally scabs over. The lesions are more common on the trunk, and there are progressive crops of lesions. The other three choices all have maculopapular rashes. Scarlet fever has a rough sandpaper-like rash that is most pronounced in skin folds, like the groin and axilla. Rubella also has a maculopapular rash that begins on the trunk and face and then spreads to the extremities. The rash on the trunk then fades. Measles, too, has a maculopapular rash that begins on the face and trunk, and progresses to the extremities. Instead of fading on the trunk as the rash of rubella does, the rash of measles coalesces on the trunk. (Ref. 30, pp. 299–300, 827)

375. C. Ten millimeters has traditionally been used to define a positive reaction, but several things must be taken into account when evaluating the size of the reaction. These include whether or not the person has received a BCG vaccine, which is administered in many countries, though not in the United States. A reaction 10 mm or greater in someone who has received the vaccine would be considered positive. Infants and elderly people, as well as those with active disease, may have an anergic or attenuated response to the vaccine, and a positive reaction for these groups may be as little as 5 mm. Anyone suspected of exposure to TB should receive a PPD or Mantoux test because there is a measured amount of PPD present in them, unlike the screening puncture tests (such as Tine tests). (Ref. 40, pp. 29–37)

376. A. The group American Indians/Eskimos is most likely to live in crowded conditions that favor the transmission of the disease. There is also evidence that there are many cases among Asians, although population counts to compare them to other groups are not available. New York, Texas, California, and South Carolina have about half the childhood cases of TB reported in the United States. (Ref. 40, p. 30)

377. A. Other symptoms include low-grade fever and recurrent or persistent pneumonia. (Ref. 40, p. 32)

378. A. The functional murmur and the bruit are also innocent murmurs, but have different characteristics. The functional murmur is usually heard in infants and young children, and is a systolic ejection murmur heard in the pulmonic area. The bruit is also an ejection murmur heard at the base that radiates to the apex; care must be taken not to confuse that with aortic stenosis. Tetralogy of Fallot is a pathological murmur that is usually associated with a ventricular septal defect and cyanosis. (Ref. 29, pp. 473, 486)

379. C. Tonic neck reflex usually is not present in newborns, but can be observed at 2 to 3 weeks of age. (Ref. 28, p. 461)

380. B. Absence seizures are almost exclusively found in children; following the attack, the person resumes his or her previous activity. Partial seizures may be simple or complex, but are focal in that they involve all or part of one side of the body. Patients with partial simple seizures do not have changes in consciousness, whereas those with complex partial seizures do. Tonic-clonic seizures (grand mal) involve loss of consciousness, jerking movements of the extremities, and loss of urinary or fecal continence. There is also a post-ictal period associated with these seizures. A partial seizure may evolve into a generalized seizure. The terms used for this question are those used for the International Classification of Seizures. (Ref. 40, pp. 446–447, 468–469)

381. C. Ethosuximide (Zarotin) is also appropriate for this seizure disorder. Phenytoin and phenobarbital are recommended for tonic-clonic and tonic disorders; Valium is reserved for status epilepticus. (Ref. 40, p. 470)

382. D. All of the evaluations listed, except cardiac enzymes, are appropriate for evaluation of a child who receives valproic acid. (Ref. 30, pp. 626–627)

383. D. Other conditions include abnormal ocular findings such as papilledema; vomiting that is persistent, increasing in frequency, or preceded by headaches; change in the headaches; diabetes insipidus; or a child with neurofibromatosis or tuberous sclerosis. (Ref. 28, p. 469)

384. B. Hirschsprung's disease results from a portion of the colon that does not have autonomic innervation. The rectal vault in a child with this disease may be empty, whereas a child with constipation may have a full rectal vault. Anal fissures in the older child may cause pain with defecation and make the child reluctant to have a bowel movement. (Ref. 28, p. 271)

385. A. Most commonly, syphilis is spread to the infant via the placenta. Other symptoms include CNS disease, chronic rhinitis, nephrotic syndrome, osteochronditis, or perichronditis. The jaundice may be primarily the direct portion of the bilirubin, rather than the indirect, which is associated with physiologic jaundice. (Refs. 28, p. 548; 30, p. 794)

386. E. The most common cause of traveler's diarrhea is *E. coli*, and it can be identified with the methods listed in all of the choices. Duodenal aspirates are usually reserved for children who have protracted diarrhea (longer than 1 to 2 weeks), fever, chills, or bloody diarrhea. (Ref. 25, p. 56)

387. D. The other three factors all occur as the newborn adapts to extrauterine life. (Ref. 25, p. 186)

388. D. All of the findings listed are associated with this condition, found primarily in children being treated in tertiary-care nurseries. (Ref. 25, p. 196)

389. E. This clinical story may describe a variety of childhood diseases including malignancy, rheumatoid disorders, and infectious diseases such as Lyme disease, osteomyelitis, and septic arthritis. (Ref. 28, pp. 557, 1250–1251)

390. A. Leukemia is the most common childhood malignancy, with about 1,500 cases diagnosed each year. It is more common in males, and the median age of diagnosis is four years. (Ref. 25, p. 557)

391. B. The undescended testis will demonstrate abnormalities of spermatogonia, as well as a narrowed tubular diameter after the age of two. Most children who do have undescended testes at birth will have descended testes by the age of three months. If not, a course of HCG or gonadotropin-releasing hormone may cause them to descend. Even if the testes do descend, the child continues to be at risk for testicular cancer, and should be periodically evaluated as well as taught techniques for self-examination. (Ref. 25, pp. 874–875)

392. D. Puberty is the most common cause of gynecomastia. Other drugs that may cause this include spironolactone, marijuana, phenothiazines, and meprobamate. Thyroid disorders and, very rarely, malignancy, may also be the etiology. (Ref. 25, p. 877)

393. A. Boys are more likely to be enuretic. It is also more likely in black children, even when socioeconomic factors are controlled. (Ref. 30, p. 148)

394. C. It is of vital importance that the child receive encouragement from both health care workers as well as his family members. (Ref. 30, pp. 150–151)

395. E. Other factors to consider include diseases of the central nervous system, diarrheal disorders that lead to incontinence, intestinal pseudoobstruction syndrome, hypothyroidism, hypercalcemia, and diseases of the intestinal smooth muscle. (Ref. 30, p. 153)

396. C. Refusal to maintain weight at the normal minimum for height is one of several criteria used to diagnose this disease by DSM III criteria. Choices A and B are other criteria, as is a disturbance in body image and the absence of an illness that would explain the weight loss. (Ref. 30, p. 203)

397. E. This kind of reaction is a type 3 allergic reaction, ie, one that causes the complement system to be activated by the formation of drug antigen-antibody complexes. Other symptoms include lymphadenopathy, fever, urticaria, arthralgia, and general malaise. (Ref. 30, pp. 223–224)

398. B. Precordial catch syndrome causes chest pain in young, healthy individuals and occurs at rest, especially with bending. The pain apparently arises from the parietal pleura, although there is no precedent event, such as respiratory illness. (Ref. 30, p. 248)

399. C. Café-au-lait spots are brown in color and are associated with neurofibromatosis. Spider nevi occur on the face and exposed parts of the body, have a central arteriole with radiating blood vessels, and are common in school-age children. Cavernous hemangiomas are dark blue in color, deep, and contain large mature blood vessels. (Ref. 30, pp. 305, 306, 310)

400. C. The lesion is usually located in the lumbosacral area of the spine. (Ref. 25, pp. 719–720)

401. B. Other factors associated with hearing loss include Apgar score of five or less at five minutes, delayed growth and development, more than 24 hours in a neonatal intensive care unit, known physical anomalies of the skull or ENT, history of maternal or neonatal infection, history of head injury at birth or later, and family history of hereditary hearing loss. (Ref. 30, p. 376)

402. B. Allergic conjunctivitis is usually recurrent and also involves chemosis (swelling) of the lids and conjunctivae. Bacterial conjunctivitis has purulent discharge with matting of the eyelids. Herpetic conjunctivitis may be subclinical or may present as follicular conjunctivitis with ulcerative lesions of the eyelids. (Ref. 30, pp. 420–421)

403. B. This infection is usually acquired by the ascending amniotic infection syndrome; it is treated with erythromycin ointment. (Ref. 30, pp. 423, 426)

404. D. The amniotic infection syndrome is also responsible for these infections. Organisms of the vagina are able to infect the amniotic membranes that usually are ruptured. The infant then inhales or ingests the contaminated fluid while still in utero, or during the birth process. (Ref. 30, pp. 424, 798–790)

405. B. Other signs include a positive Galeazzi sign. This can be done by placing the infant in a supine position, flexing the hips to 90°, and then almost completely flexing the knees. If the test is positive, the knee on the affected side will have a shortened height compared to the normal side. Another sign is the telescoping sign. If the hip is dislocated, the femoral head and shaft can be pushed back and forth when the hip is in 90° of flexion. (Ref. 30, p. 563)

406. B. The anterior fontanelle may also be depressed. (Ref. 30, p. 764)

407. B. Either normal saline or Ringer's lactate could be started because both are isotonic and would not worsen the child's electrolyte balance. Children are also prone to become hypoglycemic with stress; therefore, dextrose should also be present in the first fluids given intravenously. (Ref. 30, p. 766)

408. E. (Ref. 30, p. 793)

409. B. The most common cause is *S. pneumoniae*. (Ref. 30, pp. 795–796)

410. D. All of the other infections listed are spread by fecal–oral routes. Most frequently, this occurs among children in diapers and the caregivers who change diapers. (Ref. 30, pp. 799–800)

411. D. Erythema multiforme. (Ref. 30, pp. 262, 267, 268, 282)

412. E. Pityriasis rosea. (Ref. 30, pp. 262, 267, 268, 282)

413. A. Atopic dermatitis. (Ref. 30, pp. 262, 267, 268, 282)

414. B. Acne. (Ref. 30, pp. 262, 267, 268, 282)

415. C. Seborrheic dermatitis. (Ref. 30, pp. 262, 267, 268, 282)

9 Cardiology

DIRECTIONS (Questions 416–423): Each of the questions or incomplete statements below is followed by four or five suggested answers or completions. Select the one that is best in each case.

---

416. Which of the following statements concerning atherosclerosis is NOT true?
   A. HDL (high-density lipoprotein) elevation has been shown to be protective of ischemic heart disease
   B. Diabetes mellitus has not been shown to increase the incidence of ischemic heart disease or myocardial infarction
   C. Xanthomas are indicative of genetic disorder of lipoprotein metabolism
   D. There is evidence that it is possible to correct hyperlipidemia

417. Which of the following is NOT a predisposing pathophysiologic factor of angina pectoris?
   A. Atherosclerosis
   B. Anemia
   C. Valvular dysfunction
   D. Anxiety

143

418. Cigarette smoking has been shown to cause which of the following in its relationship to the cardiovascular system?
    A. It may result in constriction of the coronary vessels
    B. It has been shown to have no effect on blood pressure
    C. It has not been shown to have a demonstrable effect on heart rate
    D. It has been thought to help reduce HDL levels in the blood

419 Which of the following is NOT considered a therapeutic approach to patients with angina pectoris?
    A Surgery
    B. Nitroglycerin tablets
    C. Avoidance of all angina-precipitating activity
    D. Calcium channel blockers

420. The MOST reliable means of recognition of acute myocardial infarction is
    A. electrocardiogram
    B. physical exam
    C. history
    D. serum enzyme changes

421. Which of the following is the MOST common cause of aortic aneurysm?
    A. Trauma
    B. Arteriosclerosis
    C. Infection
    D. Marfan's syndrome

422. Which of the following diseases is associated with Raynaud's phenomenon?
    A. Scleroderma
    B. Buerger's disease
    C. Raynaud's disease
    D. All of the above

423. Which of the following statements concerning findings on special-
ized cardiac diagnostic tests is **FALSE?**
  A. A "water bottle" cardiac silhouette configuration is highly
  suggestive of a pericardial effusion
  B. On the standard PA and lateral radiographic views, the single
  most important cardiac observation is ventricular size
  C. Changes in the vascularization of the pulmonary bed are
  good prognosticators of cardiac disease
  D. Fluoroscopy can reveal faint calcifications in the coronary
  vessels or cardiac valves, suggestive of atherosclerosis

DIRECTIONS (Questions 424–430): For each of the questions or in-
complete statements below, **one or more** of the answers or completions
given are correct. Select:
  A if only **1, 2,** and **3** are correct,
  B if only **1** and **3** are correct,
  C if only **2** and **4** are correct,
  D if only **4** is correct,
  E if **all** are correct.

---

424. There are known major risk factors associated with increased incidence of coronary disease. Which of the following is/are **TRUE** risk
factors?
  1. Elevated cholesterol
  2. Smoking
  3. Hypertension
  4. Obesity

425. Which of the following statements concerning heart sounds is/are
CORRECT?
  1. Most third heart sounds originate in the left ventricle, are
  best heard at the apex, and do not vary with respiration
  2. Third heart sounds are more often physiologic than
  pathologic, especially in adults over 40
  3. A noncompliant ventricle most often results from
  hypertrophy or thickening in response to chronic pressure
  load, as in hypertension
  4. S-1 is the sound heard at the end of systole, when the mitral
  and tricuspid valves close

Directions Summarized				
A	B	C	D	E
1,2,3 only	1,3 only	2,4 only	4 only	All are correct

426. Which of the following statements concerning heart murmurs is/are **CORRECT?**
  1. A clinician's ability to distinguish heart murmurs and sounds of benign origin helps patients avoid unnecessary anxiety and expense
  2. An innocent murmur usually needs no further investigation
  3. Most murmurs can be accurately diagnosed by using only auscultation and bedside maneuvers
  4. The intensity of murmurs does not necessarily correlate with the severity of the lesion

427. In congestive heart failure,
  1. dyspnea is a major finding
  2. decreased cardiac output results in renin/aldosterone-induced salt and water retention
  3. compensatory mechanisms of the heart (hypertrophy and dilation) may allow the patient to perform almost normally without symptoms
  4. ventricular function is best characterized by contractility and compliance

428. Concerning the physiology of the heart, which of the following statements is/are **CORRECT?**
  1. Semilunar valve closure follows atrioventricular opening in the cardiac cycle
  2. Ventricular filling is most rapid during late diastole in the cardiac cycle
  3. The two components of the second heart sound come closer together during expiration
  4. The third heart sound is a reliable sign of myocardial disease

429. Which of the following statements is/are **TRUE** concerning the complications of acute myocardial infarction?
1. Infarct extension is an important complication; approximately 50% of patients extend their myocardial infarcts within the first five days
2. More than 90% of patients develop ventricular premature beats in the first 72 hours after acute myocardial infarction
3. Patients with cardiogenic shock as a consequence of left ventricular damage occurring in acute myocardial infarction have a good prognosis
4. Acute left bundle branch block ordinarily develops as a consequence of a large anterior myocardial infarction

430. Which of the following systemic conditions and diseases is/are **MOST** likely to exhibit cardiac manifestations?
1. Systemic hypertension
2. Thyroid disease
3. SLE
4. Cardiac amyloidosis

DIRECTIONS (Questions 431–440): The group of questions below consists of lettered headings followed by a list of numbered words, phrases, or statements. For each numbered word, phrase, or statement, select the **one** lettered heading that is most closely associated with it. Each lettered heading may be selected once, more than once, or not at all.

Questions 431–435: Match the valvular condition with the appropriate presentation.
- **A.** Aortic regurgitation
- **B.** Atrial septal defect
- **C.** Mitral stenosis
- **D.** Mitral regurgitation
- **E.** Aortic stenosis

431. Crescendo–decrescendo or ejection murmur, often associated with a thrill heard at the base of the heart and an S-4 gallop; there is also a narrow pulse pressure

432. Loud, early systolic or decrescendo diastolic murmur, radiating to the base of the heart

433. Midsystolic rumble; wide, fixed split S-2; left parasternal heave

434. Rumbling, low-pitched diastolic murmur heard best at the apex; S-1 snap and opening snap present

435. High-pitched, blowing holosystolic murmur heard best at the apex, radiating to left sternal border and left axilla

Questions 436–440: Match the EKG strips with the best answer.
   A. LVH
   B. RBBB
   C. Sinus tachycardia
   D. Artificial pacemaker
   E. LBBB

436. See Figure 3

437. See Figure 4

438. See Figure 5

439. See Figure 6

440. See Figure 7

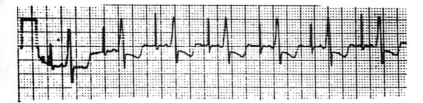

Figure 3

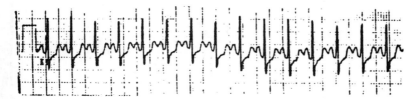

Figure 4

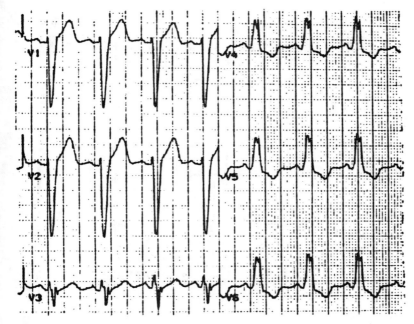

Figure 5

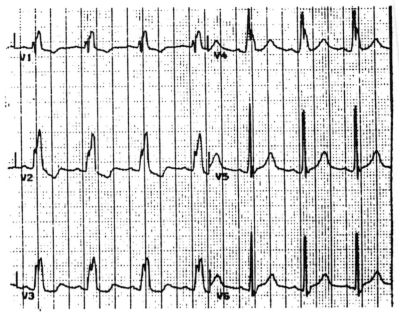

Figure 6

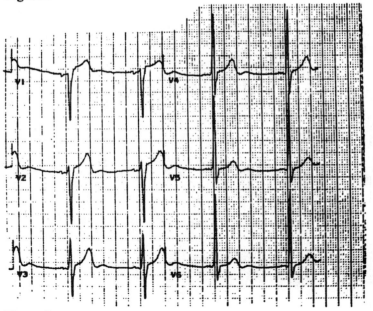

Figure 7

Explanatory Answers

416. B. Diabetes mellitus has been shown to cause a two-fold incidence in myocardial infarction. (Ref. 41, pp. 320–321)

417. D. Anxiety may coexist, but is not a physiologic factor. (Ref. 41, pp. 323–324)

418. A. Cigarette smoking increases oxygen demand, is a vasoconstrictor, increases BP, increases heart rate, and has no effect on HDL. (Ref. 41, p. 321)

419. C. Bypass surgery, vasodilators, and drugs to decrease vascular resistance are standard; nitroglycerin prophylactically allows for most normal activities. (Ref. 41, pp. 326–327)

420. C. Small infarcts may be asymptomatic, and have no changes on EKG or enzymes for hours. A good history is of the utmost importance. (Ref. 41, pp. 330–332)

421. B. Arteriosclerosis is the most common cause of aortic aneurysm. (Ref. 41, p. 370)

422. D. All of the diseases listed are causes. (Ref. 41, p. 375)

423. B. The single most important cardiac observation is heart size. (Ref. 41, pp. 192–195)

424. A. Obesity alone has not been shown to increase CAD. (Ref. 421, pp. 36–37)

425. B. Third heart sounds are more often pathologic, especially in older adults. The first heart sound is the opening of the mitral and tricuspid valves at the start of systole. (Ref. 42, p. 421)

426. E. All of the statements listed are true. (Ref. 42, pp. 43–44)

427. E. All of the statements listed are true. (Ref. 42, pp. 52–53)

428. B. Ventricular filling is most rapid during early diastole. The third heart sound is usually physiologic in children and healthy young adults. (Ref. 42, pp. 38–40)

429. C.   Only 10% extend their infarcts in the first five days; cardiogenic shock has a poor prognosis. (Ref. 41, p. 333)

430. E.   All of the conditions and diseases listed exhibit cardiac manifestations. (Ref. 41, p. 369)

431. E.   (Ref. 42, pp. 63–73)

432. A.   (Ref. 42, pp. 63–73)

433. B.   (Ref. 42, pp. 63–73)

434. C.   (Ref. 42, pp. 63–73)

435. D.   (Ref. 42, pp. 63–73)

436. D.   Artificial pacemaker. (Ref. 43, pp. 138–146)

437. C.   Sinus tachycardia. (Ref. 43, p. 48)

438. E.   LBBB. (Ref. 43, pp. 100–103)

439. B.   RBBB. (Ref. 43, p. 99)

440. A.   LVH. (Ref. 43, pp. 122–123)

10 Dermatology

DIRECTIONS (Questions 441–452): Each of the questions or incomplete statements below is followed by four or five suggested answers or completions. Select the **one** that is best in each case.

---

441. Which of the following is characteristic of basal cell carcinoma?
   A. Can be differentiated from other skin cancers by its waxy nodular rolled edges
   B. Bleeding is not a frequent finding
   C. Metastases are common
   D. Rapid growth

442. Which of the following is an acquired anomaly of the skin characterized by depigmented white patches surrounded by a normal or hyperpigmented border?
   A. Melasma
   B. Poikiloderma of Civatte
   C. Vitiligo
   D. Café-au-lait

443. Which of the following statements is **NOT** characteristic of scleroderma?
   A. Skeletal manifestations are first noted by articular pain, swelling, and inflammation
   B. The earliest changes often occur insidiously, upon the face and the hands
   C. Appearance of edema of the skin and red soft nodules
   D. Partial alopecia and decreased sweat gland activity are frequently found

444. Giant hairy nevus
   A. typically develops in the second decade of life
   B. requires total removal for the most effective treatment
   C. is not associated with malignancy
   D. usually does not exceed 3 to 4 cm in size

445. Which of the following is/are a cutaneous manifestation of SLE?
   A. Palmar and plantar surfaces of hands and feet, elbows, knees, and buttocks can develop persistant erythema or purplish discoloration
   B. Alopecia aereata
   C. Discoid patches of erythematous macules, and edema across the malar region of the face
   D. All of the above

446. A Wood's light is **NOT** helpful in the diagnosis of
   A. tinea capitus
   B. erythrasma
   C. vitiligo
   D. lichen chronicus simplex

447. Which statement is **NOT** true of malignant melanoma?
   A. Melanoma is not commonly encountered in the darker races
   B. Melanoma may simulate a wide variety of lesions
   C. The color is usually uniform throughout the tumor
   D. The diagnosis is always established by biopsy

448. The biopsy method considered **MOST** appropriate for suspected skin cancer is
   A. punch biopsy
   B. shave biopsy
   C. excisional biopsy
   D. incisional biopsy

449. Which of the following drugs is **MOST** frequently associated with photosensitivity?
   A. Penicillin
   B. Tetracycline
   C. Aspirin
   D. PABA

450. In which of the following skin disease processes would you **NOT** expect to find nail changes?
   A. Psoriasis
   B. Lichen planus
   C. Atopic dermatitis
   D. Rosacea

451. Which of the following is **NOT** a recognition feature of malignant melanoma?
   A. Asymmetry of the lesion itself
   B. Irregular borders of the lesion
   C. Continuity of color throughout
   D. Diameter greater than 6 mm before recognition

452. Which of the following is **NOT** associated with folliculitis?
   A. Staphyloccal infection
   B. *P. aeruginosa*
   C. *C. albicans*
   D. Coliforms

DIRECTIONS (Questions 453–460): For each of the questions or incomplete statements below, **one or more** of the answers or completions given are correct. Select:

    A if only **1, 2,** and **3** are correct,
    B if only **1** and **3** are correct,
    C if only **2** and **4** are correct,
    D if only **4** is correct,
    E if **all** are correct.

---

453. Treatment of hypertrophic scars may include which of the following?
    1. Intralesional corticosteroid injections
    2. Careful reexcision
    3. No treatment
    4. Electrical dessication

454. Characteristics of pityrisis rosea include
    1. an initial erythematous round lesion, 2 to 6 cm with scaly plaque appearing anywhere on the body
    2. treatment is usually not indicated
    3. pruritis may or may not be present
    4. self-limiting; thought to be viral in origin

455. The **MOST** common known causes of erythema multiforme is/are
    1. diabetes mellitus
    2. drugs
    3. hereditary factors
    4. infection

456. Useful agents in the treatment of tinea versicolor include
    1. keratolytic creams
    2. selenium sulfide suspensions
    3. miconazole, tolafinate preparations
    4. oral griseofulvin

457. Which of the following statements is/are **TRUE** of erythema nodosum?
1. Most common in young women
2. Staphyloccal infection is the most common preceding cause
3. Will subside spontaneously in 3 to 6 weeks
4. The nodule is painless

458. Which of the following is/are thought to be itiologic factors of urticaria?
1. Infection
2. Stress
3. Food allergies
4. Drugs

459. The differential diagnosis for seborrheic dermatitis includes
1. lupus erythematosis
2. psoriasis
3. tinea capitus
4. pityrisis rosea

460. Which of the following statements concerning acne vulgaris is/are **TRUE**?
1. Acne is mostly a condition found in adolescents
2. Acne is thought to be directly related to diet
3. Acne is the most common disease seen by the dermatologist
4. Acne is thought to be a function of poor hygiene

DIRECTIONS (Questions 461–465): The group of questions below consists of lettered headings followed by a list of numbered words, phrases, or statements. For each numbered word, phrase, or statement, select the **one** lettered heading that is most closely associated with it. Each lettered heading may be selected once, more than once, or not at all.

Match the disease with the description.

    A. Psoriasis
    B. Ichthyosis
    C. Chronic parapsoriasis
    D. Lichen planus
    E. Reiter's syndrome

461. Violaceous, polygonal, flat-topped papules; Wickam's striae often on wrist and ankles, associated with Koebner reaction

462. Erythematous silvery scaled plaques; hyperkeratotic papules of palms and soles; frequently involves mouth and genitals. Distribution involves elbows, knees, and scalp

463. A variety of syndromes with variation of scaling from fine to large, thick scales, involving flexor and extensor surfaces

464. Erythematous plaques with silvery mica-like scales; usually nonpruritic; nail involvement with wide distribution

465. Guttate to larger, red scaling papules and plaques; nonpruritic

Explanatory Answers

441. A. Rapid growth and metastases are not common in basal cell carcinomas; bleeding is frequently found; waxy rolled edges is the common presentation. (Ref. 46, pp. 763–764)

442. C. Melasma is a hyperpigmented condition; poikiloderma of Civatte reticulated, red-brown condition; vitiligo is the depigmented condition; café-au-lait seen in von Recklinghausen's disease. (Ref. 46, p. 1000)

443. C. Skin is taut, bound down, and the lesions are ivory or yellow under the skin—not red or edematous. (Ref. 46, pp. 176–178)

444. B. Giant hairy nevi are usually present at birth, are associated with malignant melanoma, and may cover large areas, typically the trunk. Total removal is recommended to reduce the chance of cancer. (Ref. 46, pp. 815–816)

445. D. All of the choices listed can be cutaneous manifestations of SLE. (Ref. 46, p. 167)

446. D. All of the choices fluoresce except lichen chronicus simplex, which is a chronic dermatitis. (Ref. 46, p. 18)

447. C. The color varies in shades; melanoma can appear as other lesions; biopsy is important in making the diagnosis; and melanoma usually is not seen in dark skin races. (Ref. 46, pp. 819–822)

448. C. Complete removal with margins is the preferred method in suspected cancer, especially in malignant melanoma. (Ref. 41, p. 2313)

449. B. Tetracycline is one of the systemic sensitizers, penicillin is not. Aspirin is a prostaglandin inhibitor and may protect against the sun; PABA is used in sunscreens to block UV rays. (Ref. 41, p. 2330)

450. D. Psoriasis causes pitting of nails; lichen planus can cause ridging; atopic dermatitis can cause pitting striations and onycholysis. Rosacea is associated with acne. (Ref. 41, pp. 2346–2347)

451. C. The basics of melanoma recognition are important to learn. The color of melanoma characteristically varies in shades due to the depth of cancerous invasion of the skin. (Ref. 41, p. 2338)

452. D. All of the above except coliforms, which resemble *E. coli*, are associated with folliculitis. They are not skin infectives. (Ref. 41, p. 2334)

453. A. Electrical dessication increases scarring. (Ref. 44, p. 140)

454. E. All of the characteristics listed are a typical presentation. (Ref. 44, p. 154)

455. C. Sulfonamides and herpes simplex infections are the most frequent cause. (Ref. 45, pp. 79–82)

456. A. Oral antifungals are of no use. (Ref. 45, p. 101)

457. B. Self-resolving and common in women, strep infection is most common; the nodule is painful. (Ref. 45, pp. 193–194)

458. E. All of the choices listed are factors of urticaria. (Ref. 45, p. 197)

459. A. The first three choices are scaley, erythematous; pityrisis rosea distribution is not correct. (Ref. 45, p. 107)

460. B. Diet and hygiene have been proven false as precipitating factors. (Ref. 46, pp. 250–257)

461. D. These are classic presentations. (Ref. 41, p. 2326)

462. E. (Ref. 41, p. 2326)

463. B. (Ref. 41, p. 2326)

464. A. (Ref. 41, p. 2326)

465. C. (Ref. 41, p. 2326)

11 Gastrointestinal System

DIRECTIONS (Questions 466–482): Each of the questions or incomplete statements below is followed by four or five suggested answers or completions. Select the **one** that is best in each case.

466. Which of the following treatments for gastroesophageal reflux is **NOT** considered appropriate?
- **A.** H₂ receptor blocking agents
- **B.** Liquid antacids
- **C.** Anticholinergic agents
- **D.** Antireflux surgery

467. Which of the following is considered appropriate treatment for acute pancreatitis?
- **A.** Nasogastric suction
- **B.** Anticholinergics
- **C.** Meperidine
- **D.** Antibiotic

468. Which of the following is **NOT** considered a complication of gastroesophageal reflux?
- **A.** Esophageal ulcer
- **B.** Esophageal strictures
- **C.** Pulmonary aspiration
- **D.** Esophageal varices

469. The etiology of acute gastritis includes all of the following **EXCEPT**
    A. infection
    B. drugs
    C. stress
    D. endocrine disorders

470. Which of the following statements concerning Zollinger-Ellison syndrome is **NOT** true?
    A. The pain of peptic ulcer disease is a major finding
    B. Diarrhea results almost exclusively from the large volume of fluids secreted by the stomach
    C. Neoplasm is rarely associated with this syndrome
    D. Cushing's disease may develop as a result of ACTH-secreting gastrinomas

471. The key features of irritable bowel syndrome include all of the following **EXCEPT**
    A. abdominal discomfort
    B. bleeding
    C. alterations of bowel habit
    D. frequent lack of associated organic cause

472. The increased prevalence of colorectal cancer in developed western countries may imply
    A. Asian and African cultures do not have a genetic disposition for the disease
    B. increased levels of parasitic infection in underdeveloped countries may provide some protection
    C. a direct association between increased animal fat and lack of fiber intake
    D. none of the above

473. Narrowing of the lumen of the colon may be suggestive of which of the following conditions?
    A. Diverticulitis
    B. Crohn's disease
    C. Carcinoma
    D. All of the above

474. Which of the following drugs is usually **NOT** associated with liver disease?
     A. Chlorpromazine
     B. Acetaminophen
     C. INH
     D. None of the above

475. A 45-year-old asymptomatic male was found to have gallstones on a routine exam. Which of the following statements is **TRUE**?
     A. A cholecystectomy performed now would increase the patient's lifespan
     B. There is a higher incidence of neoplasm in gallbladders with stones than in those without stones
     C. There is greater than a 50% chance that symptoms due to gallstones will develop in the future
     D. None of the above

476. In a 40-year-old alcoholic male who has had no prior complaint of abdominal pain, hematemesis is **MOST** likely due to which of the following?
     A. Peptic ulcer
     B. Diffuse hemorrhagic gastritis
     C. Bleeding esophageal varices
     D. Reflux esophagitis

477. In the previous patient, the emergency treatment would include all of the following **EXCEPT**
     A. vasopressin
     B. packed red cells and fresh frozen plasma
     C. surgical intervention
     D. nitroglycerin

478. Which of the following statements is **TRUE** of abdominal pain?
     A. Colicky-type pain only occurs when there is an intestinal obstruction
     B. Abdominal wall rigidity is a reflex spasm secondary to inflammation of the underlying peritoneum
     C. Pleuritic pain excludes a possibility of intraabdominal cause
     D. Vascular occlusion of the mesentery artery is the most common cause of intestinal ischemic pain

479. The acid concentration of the stomach is **NOT** related to which of the following factors?
    A. The speed of acid secretion
    B. Rate of duodenal emptying
    C. Buffering capacity of ingested contents
    D. Rate of gastric emptying

480. Radiographic contrast studies are useful in
    A. differentiating benign from malignant gastric ulcers
    B. defining mucosal disease of the stomach
    C. their ability to define complete healing of an ulcer
    D. none of the above

481. Following appropriate treatment, failure of ulcer symptoms to resolve is indicative of
    A. something unusual, as most patients with ulcers do respond to medical regimen
    B. possible malignancy
    C. noncompliance of the regimen
    D. all of the above

482. When large bowel bleeding is suspected, which of the following procedures should be **FIRST** employed?
    A. Angiography
    B. Fiberoptic endoscope
    C. Proctosigmoidoscopy
    D. Barium studies

DIRECTIONS (Questions 483–490): The group of questions below consists of lettered headings followed by a list of numbered words, phrases, or statements. For each numbered word, phrase, or statement, select the **one** lettered heading that is most closely associated with it. Each lettered heading may be selected once, more than once, or not at all.

Questions 483–486: Match each of the physical findings listed with an associated potential cause of gastrointestinal bleeding.

    A. Peptic ulcer
    B. Small bowel polyps
    C. Thrombocytopenia
    D. Esophageal varices

483. Melanin spots on buccal mucosa

484. Petechiae

485. Spider angiomas

486. Epigastric tenderness

Questions 487–490: Match the lettered and numbered items.

    A. Peptic ulcer disease
    B. Acute viral gastroenteritis
    C. Crohn's disease
    D. Acute pancreatitis
    E. Dissecting aortic aneurysm
    F. Giardiasis
    G. Acute cholecystitis
    H. Acute bowel obstruction

487. Steady knife-like, epigastric abdominal pain, which characteristically radiates to the left quadrant and back; vomiting is frequent

488. Right upper abdominal pain which increases gradually in severity; pain may refer to the back and may occur at the level of the scapula

489. Periumbilical episodic pain, usually postprandial, occurring in young adults; pain is frequently accompanied by low-grade fever and diarrhea

490. Intermittent epigastric burning pain; relieved with food or alkali

Explanatory Answers

466. C. Anticholinergics cause relaxation of E-G sphincter and increase reflux. (Ref. 41, p. 682)

467. C. The objective is symptomatic pain relief. All other treatments listed have been found to be of no value. (Ref. 41, p. 777)

468. D. The effect of gastric acids on the mucosa of the esophagus will cause all of the above except varices, which are related to alcohol. (Ref. 41, p. 682)

469. D. *Streptococcus* and *Campylobacter,* nonsteroidal anti-inflammatories, stress of major illness such as sepsis, or trauma may be found. Endocrine disorders may play a part in chronic gastritis. (Ref. 41, pp. 689–690)

470. C. Abdominal pain, diarrhea, and steatorrhea are common. Neoplasm (gastrinomas) occur in patients. (Ref. 41, pp. 708–709)

471. B. Bleeding is not a factor unless hemorrhoids are present. (Ref. 41, p. 722)

472. C. Increased fiber in the diet increases motility in the bowel, decreasing contact time of carcinogens. Migrants to developed nations have been found to assume the risk of the local population. (Ref. 41, p. 768)

473. D. All of the above conditions may cause some degree of narrowing or obstruction of the colon. (Ref. 41, p. 804)

474. D. All of the drugs listed have been shown to be associated with liver toxicity. (Ref. 41, pp. 828–829)

475. B. Cholecystectomy in an asymptomatic patient has not shown to increase lifespan; with stones there is a 70% to 80 % increase in cancer. There is no proof that symptoms will develop in the future. (Ref. 41, pp. 863, 870)

476. C. Lack of prior abdominal pain would lead one more to consider esophageal varices. (Ref. 42, pp. 808–809)

477. D. Hypovolemia needs to be corrected. Vasopressin decreases portal flow and causes vasoconstriction of splanchnic arteries. Surgery is a last resort, and has a 50% mortality rate. Nitroglycerin would dilate vasculature and increase bleeding. (Ref. 42, pp. 809–810)

478. B. Colic-type pain is frequently, but not only, associated with obstruction. Peritoneal inflammation causes reflex abdominal wall rigidity. When an underlying inflamed organ comes into contact with the diaphragm, pleuritic-type pain is possible. Right-sided heart failure (low cardiac output) is the most common cause of intestinal ischemic pain. (Ref. 42, p. 788)

479. B. The speed of secretion, the buffering capacity of what is ingested, and the speed with which it is emptied from the stomach are important in designing appropriate therapy. (Ref. 42, p. 799)

480. D. All of the following are shortcomings of radiographic barium studies because they are not able to define mucosal disease, assure healing, or differentiate malignancy in gastric ulcers. (Ref. 42, p. 798)

481. D. With H_2 receptor antagonists, effective treatment is improved. Unhealed ulcers should be a cause for investigation. There is a need to rule-out malignancy. Noncompliance is always a consideration. (Ref. 42, p. 803)

482. C. Proctosigmoidoscopy provides better direct visualization of the mucosa of the rectum, with easier clearing of blood than the endoscope. Angiography is more invasive, but is useful if direct visualization fails. Barium studies are of no value, and may even hinder further identification of the cause of hemorrhage. (Ref. 42, p. 808)

483. B. (Ref. 42, pp. 799–805)

484. C. (Ref. 42, p. 370)

485. D. (Ref. 42, p. 342)

486. A. (Ref. 42, pp. 807–810)

487. D. (Ref. 41, p. 76)

488. G.   (Ref. 41, p. 865)

489. C.   (Ref. 41, p. 747)

490. A.   (Ref. 41, p. 695)

12 Obstetrics and Gynecology

DIRECTIONS (Questions 491–553): Each of the questions or incomplete statements below is followed by four or five suggested answers or completions. Select the **one** that is best in each case.

---

491. Vulva lesions can be due to several etiologies. An indurated, painless, well-defined ulcer with an indurated rim, accompanied by enlarged groin lymph nodes, would be **MOST** suggestive of which of the following?
    A. Granuloma inguinale
    B. Primary syphilis chancre
    C. Condyloma acuminatum
    D. Herpes virus

492. The **BEST** diagnostic test for syphilis would be one which has a low incidence of false positives, such as
    A. RPR
    B. VDRL
    C. FTA-ABS
    D. culture of syphilitic chancre
    E. CRP

493. A female patient complains of vaginal irritation and presents with frothy, greenish vaginal discharge, accompanied by "strawberry spots" on the vaginal epithelium. The clinician should be **MOST** suspicious of which of the following?

A. *C. trachomatis*
B. *C. albicans*
C. *Herpesvirus hominis*
D. *Trichomonas vaginalis*
E. *G. vaginalis*

494. A female patient presents with vaginal erythema and a thick, watery, grey discharge. "Clue cells" are noted on examination of a saline vaginal secretion smear, suggestive of which of the following?

A. *T. vaginalis*
B. *N. gonorrhea*
C. *C. albicans*
D. *S. aureus*
E. *G. vaginalis*

495. A patient being treated for a tuboovarian abscess complains of increased pelvic pain and has chills, an elevation of fever, tachycardia, and hypotension. The **BEST** treatment would be

A. observation
B. hysterectomy
C. increased antibiotics
D. semi-Fowler position

496. The incidence of ovarian cancer in the U. S. population is quite high. Risk factors include all of the following **EXCEPT**

A. high-fat diet
B. multiparity of six or greater
C. smoking
D. history of breast cancer

497. Polycystic ovary syndrome increases the risk of a patient developing

A. theca lutein cysts
B. adnexal torsion
C. corpus luteum cysts
D. endometrial adenocarcinoma

498. The majority of breast cancer is noted by the patient first detecting a lump in what location of the breast?
   A. Upper outer quadrant
   B. Upper inner quadrant
   C. Lower outer quadrant
   D. Lower inner quadrant

499. Patient education regarding self breast examination is key for early lump detection. The **BEST** time to check the breast for masses is
   A. 2 to 3 days before menses
   B. at midcycle (ovulation)
   C. during menses
   D. 2 to 3 days after menses

500. Mammography is a valuable diagnostic tool for breast cancer detection. The American Cancer Society recommends that asymptomatic women should have a baseline mammogram at what age?
   A. 20 to 25 years
   B. 25 to 30 years
   C. 35 to 40 years
   D. 45 to 50 years

501. Many laboratories continue to provide Pap smear results with the older numerical classification, as opposed to relating whether there are cells compatible with dysplasia. A patient with a class III (moderate dysplasia) Pap smear should have which of the following **NEXT** in her evaluation?
   A. Cold-knife conization
   B. Observation only
   C. Colposcopy
   D. Repeat Pap smear in six months

502. During the culdocentesis procedure, a needle is inserted into the
   A. anterior fornix
   B. posterior fornix
   C. cervical os
   D. urethra

503. Cyanosis and softening of the cervix at approximately 6 to 8 weeks gestation is termed
   A. McDonald's sign
   B. Hegar's sign
   C. Ladin's sign
   D. Goodell's sign

504. During pregnancy, when the cervix may be flexed upon the corpus, which sign is said to be present?
   A. McDonald's sign
   B. Hegar's sign
   C. Ladin's sign
   D. Goodell's sign

505. A fingertip softening of the isthmus of the cervix, suggestive of pregnancy, is called
   A. McDonald's sign
   B. Hegar's sign
   C. Ladin's sign
   D. Goodell's sign

506. Softening of the entire isthmus of the uterus transversely occurs at approximately eight weeks of gestation, and is termed
   A. McDonald's sign
   B. Hegar's sign
   C. Ladin's sign
   D. Goodell's sign

507. Normal hormonal changes associated with pregnancy can cause the clinician confusion in interpreting other lab studies. For instance, during pregnancy the thyroid gland enlarges. Thyroid lab results consistent with pregnancy are
   A. elevated TBG, decreased T3RU, normal free T4
   B. depressed TBG, decreased T3RU, normal free T4
   C. depressed TBG, increased T3RU, increased free T4
   D. elevated TBG, increased T3RU, increased free T4

508. The use of ultrasound has enabled the clinician to detect fetal presence at an earlier time than in the past. At what gestational point are fetal heart tones **FIRST** detectable using this method?
A. Day 10
B. Day 18
C. Day 28
D. Day 35
E. Day 44

509. A patient states that the last day of her last menstrual period was February 1, 1991. Using Nagele's rule, what would be her estimated date of confinement?
A. November 1, 1991
B. November 8, 1991
C. October 30, 1991
D. October 21, 1991

510. Intrauterine growth retardation becomes suspect when the measurement of fundal height falls below what percentile at what week?
A. 25th percentile, 20th week
B. 50th percentile, any week
C. 25th percentile, tenth week
D. 30th percentile, 25th week
E. Tenth percentile, any week

511. Active labor typically begins only after the cervix has dilated to which of the following degrees?
A. 2 cm
B. 3 cm
C. 6 cm
D. 7 cm
E. 10 cm

512. The time period from complete dilatation of the cervix to the delivery of the infant is called
A. prelabor
B. first stage of labor
C. second stage of labor
D. third stage of labor
E. fourth stage of labor

513. Terminology used in determining fetal station during labor will vary based on the method used at the clinical site. Most agree, however, that the term used to describe the level of the ischial spines is
A. −3 station
B. −2 station
C. −1 station
D. 0 station
E. 1 station

514. If pain relief during labor is to be achieved with medication, care must be taken to choose a drug and route of administration that results in relief of maternal pain or agitation with little fetal effect. The **BEST** single choice is
A. promethazine hydrochloride (Phenergan) IM
B. promethazine hydrochloride (Phenergan) IV
C. hydroxyzine hydrochloride (Vistaril), IV
D. meperidine hydrochloride (Demerol), IM
E. meperidine hydrochloride (Demerol), IV

515. In considering delivery anesthesia, it is helpful to recall the sensory innervation of the lower vagina and pelvic floor. These sensory paths derive from which of the following?
A. T4-T6
B. T10-L1
C. T11-T12
D. L1-S1
E. S2-S4

516. One route of sensory anesthesia during labor is to inject anesthetic solution by way of a needle inside the vagina, over the sacrospinous ligament. The route described is used for which block?
A. Local block
B. Epidural block
C. Paracervical block
D. Pudendal block
E. Caudal block

517. Immediately after delivery, the vagina and cervix should be examined for lacerations. Which of the following terms describes a vaginal laceration that involves the superficial and deep tissue as well as the rectal sphincter?
A. First-degree laceration
B. Second-degree laceration
C. Third-degree laceration
D. Fourth-degree laceration
E. Incomplete laceration

518. A postdelivery vaginal laceration that involves superficial and deep tissue, but **NOT** the rectal sphincter, is called
A. first-degree laceration
B. second-degree laceration
C. third-degree laceration
D. fourth-degree laceration
E. fifth-degree laceration

519. All of the following are components of the Apgar score **EXCEPT**
A. appearance
B. grimace
C. respiration
D. weight
E. pulse

520. A newborn is pink, has a pulse of 80, cries spontaneously, but is gasping with hypoventilation noted, and has good movement. His Apgar score based on these characteristics is which of the following?
A. 10
B. 8
C. 6
D. 5
E. 2

521. In determining intrauterine growth retardation, the relationship of the fetal head circumference to the fetal abdominal circumference is helpful. Which of the following **BEST** reflects the ratio relationship of head circumference to abdominal circumference?
   A. >1.0 prior to 32 weeks
   B. >1.0 at all times
   C. <1.0 at all times
   D. <1.0 at 32 weeks
   E. 1.0 at all times

522. A patient in her 15th week of pregnancy presents with vaginal bleeding and lower abdominal cramps. Her membranes are intact and the cervix is closed. Which term below **BEST** applies to this patient's condition?
   A. Missed abortion
   B. Threatened abortion
   C. Inevitable abortion
   D. Incomplete abortion
   E. Habitual abortion

523. A 16-week pregnant patient presents with vaginal bleeding, cramping, a dilated cervix, but no passage of fetal tissue. Her condition is **BEST** described by which of the following terms?
   A. Missed abortion
   B. Threatened abortion
   C. Inevitable abortion
   D. Incomplete abortion
   E. Habitual abortion

524. A patient presents in the latter part of her first trimester. Her uterus is not growing appropriately for gestational age. Ultrasound indicates an indistinct gestational sac and no fetal heartbeat. Which of the following terms may describe this patient's condition?
   A. Missed abortion
   B. Threatened abortion
   C. Inevitable abortion
   D. Incomplete abortion
   E. Habitual abortion

525. Drugs, alcohol, and cigarette smoking all affect fetal growth and development. At what point in the pregnancy does the smoking of cigarettes have its **MAJOR** effect?
A. First month
B. First trimester
C. Second trimester
D. Last four months
E. Last month

526. Which organism should be highly suspected in a patient with post-partum endometriosis with fever occurring within the first 24 hours?
A. *E. coli*
B. Group B *Streptococcus*
C. Group A *Streptococcus*
D. *Proteus* species
E. *Clostridia* species

527. A patient in her seventh month of pregnancy presents after a high-impact auto accident. She has painful vaginal bleeding and a tender uterus. Which of the following should be highly suspect in your mind?
A. Placenta previa
B. Tuboovarian abscess
C. Ruptured uterus
D. Abruptio placenta
E. Incompetent cervix

528. Placenta previa can be low lying, partial, or total. Regardless, treatment usually is determined based upon the gestational age of the fetus. Delivery or C-section is the recommended course after what gestational age?
A. 26
B. 28
C. 30
D. 34
E. 37

529. The differentiating factor between a diagnosis of eclampsia versus preeclampsia is the presence of which one of the following?
   A. Hypertension
   B. Convulsions
   C. Proteinuria
   D. Oliguria
   E. Edema

530. Pregnancy-induced hypertension (PIH), a relatively new term used to include patients with eclampsia and preeclampsia, is treated by which of the following prior to delivery?
   A. Magnesium sulfate
   B. Calcium gluconate
   C. Potassium chloride
   D. Sodium bicarbonate
   E. Phosphoric acid

531. Which of the following is a candidate for Rho (D) immune globulin?
   A. Rh⁻ mother with previous abortion
   B. Rh⁺ mother with previous abortion
   C. Rh⁻ mother with previous Rh⁻ infant
   D. Rh⁺ mother with previous Rh⁻ infant
   E. Rh⁺ mother previously given Rho immune globulin

532. All of the following would be a normal baseline fetal heart rate (FHR) **EXCEPT**
   A. 180
   B. 160
   C. 150
   D. 140
   E. 130

533. A fetal monitor deceleration pattern which is abrupt in onset and abrupt in return to its baseline, with either a V-shaped, W-shaped, or U-shaped pattern, is characteristic of which of the following causes?
   A. Fetal health
   B. Cord compression
   C. Uteroplacental insufficiency
   D. Head compression
   E. Fetal anemia

534. A fetal monitor pattern that indicates smooth decelerations which start after the uterine contraction begins and persist beyond the contraction is characteristic of which of the following?
   A. Uteroplacental insufficiency
   B. Cord compression
   C. Head compression
   D. Normal labor pattern
   E. Fetal anemia

535. Several drugs are used to treat premature labor. Which one of the following drugs is the only one approved by the FDA for this purpose?
   A. Diazoxide
   B. Isoxsuprine hydrochloride
   C. Terbutaline sulfate
   D. Ritodrine hydrochloride
   E. Magnesium sulfate

536. All patients with premature rupture of the membranes should be evaluated for the presence of which of the following organisms associated with fetal deaths in premature infants?
   A. Group B streptococci
   B. *H. influenzae*
   C. *Proteus* species
   D. *Clostridia* species
   E. *E. coli*

537. Which term applies to a fetus delivered before 38 weeks gestation?
   A. Postdated fetus
   B. Predated fetus
   C. Premature fetus
   D. Term fetus
   E. Postmature fetus

538. Which of the following is used to describe the fetal position in which the hips are flexed and the knees extended so that the legs come to lie alongside fetal head?
A. Complete breech
B. Full breach
C. Incomplete breech
D. Frank breech
E. Double footling presentation

539. To decrease the risk of uterine rupture and maternal death, which of the following presentations, if detected in labor, is an indication for a cesarean section?
A. Occiput posterior presentation
B. Occiput anterior presentation
C. Brow presentation
D. Shoulder presentation
E. Face presentation

540. After delivery, if the placenta does not deliver, it may need to be removed manually. Which of the following terms describes the condition in which the placenta is attached to the myometrium of the uterus?
A. Placenta previa
B. Placenta abruptio
C. Placenta increta
D. Placenta percreta
E. Placenta accreta

541. Which of the following terms is used to describe the condition in which the placenta actually invades deeply into the myometrium?
A. Placenta previa
B. Placenta abruptio
C. Placenta increta
D. Placenta percreta
E. Placenta accreta

542. Which of the following terms describes the condition in which the placenta penetrates through the myometrium to the peritoneal surface of the uterus?
   A. Placenta previa
   B. Placenta abruptio
   C. Placenta increta
   D. Placenta percreta
   E. Placenta accreta

543. A 36-year-old female presents complaining of dry, itchy areas around the nipple of her left breast. Upon examination, the nipple and surrounding areolar area is covered by an eczematoid weeping lesion. No nipple discharge is noted. Your recommendation to this patient should be which of the following?
   A. Topical steroids
   B. Chemotherapy
   C. Radiation
   D. Nipple biopsy

544. A 50-year-old female presents complaining of urinary frequency and urgency. Upon physical, it is noted that when the patient strains, the anterior vaginal wall bulges while the posterior wall is depressed by the speculum. The history and findings suggest which of the following?
   A. Cystocele
   B. Rectocele
   C. Urethrocele
   D. Prolapsed uterus

545. Even healthy women need nutritional changes during pregnancy. Which of the following should be increased in all pregnant women?
   A. Magnesium
   B. Phosphate
   C. Sodium
   D. Iron
   E. Vitamin B_{12}

546. A 35-year-old nongravid patient presents with menorrhagia and shortened intervals between menses. She is a candidate for which procedure?

A. Laparoscopy
B. Dilatation and curettage
C. Dilatation and evacuation
D. Curettage and evacuation
E. Hysteroscopy

547. Some postmenopausal women become mildly hirsute. This is due to which mechanism below?

A. Decreased estrogen, increased LH, increased testosterone
B. Decreased estrogen, decreased LH, increased testosterone
C. Increased estrogen, decreased LH, increased testosterone
D. Increased estrogen, decreased LH, decreased testosterone
E. Decreased estrogen, decreased LH, decreased testosterone

548. The **MOST** common cause of a spontaneous abortion in the first trimester is which of the following?

A. Abnormal product of conception
B. Infection
C. Incompetent cervix
D. Uterine dysfunction
E. Diabetes mellitus

549. The average amount of blood lost during a typical menstrual cycle is which of the following?

A. 10 mL
B. 20 mL
C. 30 mL
D. 80 mL
E. 100 mL

550. A patient presents complaining of frequent periods. She is having
   A. menorrhagia
   B. metrorrhagia
   C. oligomenorrhea
   D. amenorrhea
   E. polymenorrhea

551. A patient presents complaining that her menstrual periods are decreasing in frequency. She has
   A. menorrhagia
   B. metrorrhagia
   C. oligomenorrhea
   D. amenorrhea
   E. polymenorrhea

552. A patient presents because she has started to bleed in between her periods. She has
   A. menorrhagia
   B. metrorrhagia
   C. oligomenorrhea
   D. amenorrhea
   E. polymenorrhea

553. A patient complains that her periods have recently become extremely heavy. She has
   A. menorrhagia
   B. metrorrhagia
   C. oligomenorrhea
   D. amenorrhea
   E. polymenorrhea

DIRECTIONS (Questions 554–586): For each of the questions or incomplete statements below, **one or more** of the answers or completions given are correct. Select:

    A   if only **1, 2,** and **3** are correct,
    B   if only **1** and **3** are correct,
    C   if only **2** and **4** are correct,
    D   if only **4** is correct,
    E   if **all** are correct.

---

554. The use of KOH in examining a vaginal secretion/discharge can aid the diagnosis of which of the following conditions?
1. Monilial vaginitis
2. *Trichomonas* vaginitis
3. *Gardnerella* vaginitis
4. *C. trachomatis*

555. Metronidazole (Flagyl) is used in treating which of the following vaginal infections?
1. *C. albicans*
2. *G. vaginalis*
3. *C. trachomatis*
4. *T. vaginalis*

556. Causative agents for acute cervicitis include which of the following?
1. *G. vaginalis*
2. *C. trachomatis*
3. *C. albicans*
4. *N. gonorrhoeae*

557. Causes of secondary dysmenorrhea include
1. endometriosis
2. ovarian cysts
3. uterine polyps
4. pelvic infections

Directions Summarized				
A	**B**	**C**	**D**	**E**
1,2,3	1,3	2,4	4	All are
only	only	only	only	correct

558. Risk factors for development of cervical cancer include
1. early sexual exposure
2. low parity
3. multiple sexual partners
4. advanced age

559. A patient presents complaining of dysuria and purulent vaginal discharge. You suspect acute salpingo-oophoritis and would expect to find which of the following on physical examination?
1. Elevated temperature
2. Tender adnexal regions
3. Tender cervix
4. Palpable mass

560. Signs and symptoms associated with endometriosis include
1. dysmenorrhea
2. dyspareunia
3. low backache near menses
4. menorrhagia

561. Therapy for endometriosis varies according to the severity of the patient's symptoms, her age, and interest in childbearing. Hormonal treatment to suppress ovulation and menstruation can be accomplished using which of the following?
1. Diethylstilbestrol
2. Medroxyprogesterone
3. Danazol
4. Methyltestosterone

562. Stein-Levanthal syndrome is associated with which of the following?
1. Anovulation
2. Menorrhagia
3. Infertility
4. Cachexia

563. Risk factors associated with breast cancer include
1. early menarche
2. fatty diet
3. late menopause
4. increased parity

564. Not all clinicians will agree that three samples should be taken for a Pap smear, or even what should be the sampling sites. For proper cytopathological diagnosis, endocervical cells are essential. To assure that such cells are present, which of the following sites must be sampled?
1. Vaginal pool
2. Squamocolumnar junction
3. Vaginal wall
4. Endocervical

565. Culdocentesis is a useful diagnostic procedure in patients with which of the following?
1. Ectopic pregnancy
2. Ovarian carcinoma
3. Tuboovarian abscess
4. Abnormal Pap smear

566. Which of the following should **NOT** be performed on the pregnant patient?
1. Endometrial biopsy
2. Pap smear
3. Hysteroscopy
4. Culdocentesis

567. A positive diagnosis of pregnancy can be made based upon which of the following?
1. Fetal heart tone detection
2. Positive pregnancy test
3. Fetal palpation
4. Linea nigra

	Directions Summarized			
A	**B**	**C**	**D**	**E**
1,2,3	1,3	2,4	4	All are
only	only	only	only	correct

568. The estimated date of confinement (EDC) can be calculated using Nagele's rule. The calculation is reflected in which choice below?
   1. Last day of LMP + 7 days − 3 months
   2. First day of LMP + 280 days
   3. First day of LMP + 9 months + 7 days
   4. Last day of LMP + 10 days − 2 months

569. The pain associated with uterine contractions during labor can be relieved either partially or completely by
   1. local block
   2. paracervical block
   3. pudendal block
   4. epidural block

570. Risks associated with epidural or caudal blocks include
   1. inadvertent spinal anesthesia
   2. hypotension
   3. systemic toxicity
   4. delayed labor

571. Amniocentesis is a very useful procedure in modern obstetrical procedures. Although fetal risks are rare, they do exist. Which of the following are potential fetal risks?
   1. Hemorrhage
   2. Premature labor
   3. Infection
   4. Death

572. Several tests can be used in the trimester to assess "fetal reserve" and jeopardy. Which of the following tests can be used in this assessment?
   1. Oxytocin challenge test (OCT)
   2. Nipple stimulation test
   3. Nonstress test (NST)
   4. L/S ratio

573. Patients predisposed to ectopic pregnancies are those with which of the following?
1. Pelvic inflammatory disease
2. Salpingostomy
3. Previous ectopic pregnancy
4. Tubal ligation

574. Symptoms classically associated with an ectopic pregnancy include
1. amenorrhea
2. vaginal bleeding
3. pain
4. headache

575. A 25-year-old female presents with lower right abdominal pain, nausea, weakness, tachycardia, and a fever of 39.4 °C. Her LMP was eight weeks ago. Which of the following should be included in her differential diagnosis?
1. PID
2. Appendicitis
3. Ectopic pregnancy
4. Tuboovarian abscess

576. A 20-year-old female patient presents with lower right abdominal pain, nausea, and weakness. Her LMP was ten weeks previous. The pelvic exam reveals severe tenderness upon movement of the cervix. The patient is afebrile. Which of the following should be included in the diagnostic possibilities?
1. Ectopic pregnancy
2. Threatened abortion
3. Fallopian tube torsion
4. Ruptured corpus luteum cyst

577. Due to the fetal damage that can be caused during pregnancy by certain infections, which of the following should **NOT** be administered during pregnancy?
1. Killed vaccines
2. Toxoids
3. Immunoglobulin preparations
4. Live vaccines

Directions Summarized				
A	**B**	**C**	**D**	**E**
1,2,3	1,3	2,4	4	All are
only	only	only	only	correct

578. A pregnant patient with which of the following should be evaluated for diabetes?
    1. Hydramnios
    2. History of babies over nine pounds
    3. Persistent monilial vulvoaginitis
    4. Previous unexplained stillbirth

579. Which of the following are acceptable methods of treating hyperthyroidism diagnosed during pregnancy?
    1. Propilthiouracil (PTU)
    2. Surgery
    3. Methimazole (Tapazole)
    4. ^{131}I ablation therapy

580. An incompetent cervix can lead to premature deliveries. Which of the following are etiologic factors associated with an incompetent cervix?
    1. Bicornuate uterus
    2. Cervical conization
    3. Septate uterus
    4. Functional impairment

581. Cervical cerclage is the primary treatment of an incompetent cervix. Contraindications to this include which of the following?
    1. Uterine bleeding
    2. Ruptured membranes
    3. Uterine contractions
    4. Chorioamnionitis

582. A fetal monitor pattern that has smooth decelerations which begin and end at the same time of the contractions indicates which of the following?
    1. Severe fetal distress
    2. Early deceleration
    3. Cord compression
    4. Head compression pattern

583. Fetal monitor baseline variability may be caused by which of the following?
1. Prematurity
2. Fetal hypoxia
3. Sleeping fetus
4. Thyroid medication

584. Which of the following is suggestive of cephalopelvic disproportion?
1. Fetal head molding
2. Frank breech presentation
3. Caput formation
4. Fetal hydrocephalus

585. Drugs used to suppress lactation include which of the following?
1. Chlorotrianisene (Tace)
2. Diethylstilbestrol
3. Bromocriptine (Parlodel)
4. Ethynyl estradiol

586. With the advent of the "low-dose birth control pills," some previous contraindications are being reconsidered and may no longer apply. Patients with which of the following, however, should still **NOT** receive oral contraceptives?
1. Depression
2. Headaches
3. Cigarette smoking
4. Thrombophlebitis

DIRECTIONS (Questions 587–590): Each of the questions or incomplete statements below is followed by four or five suggested answers or completions. Select the **one** that is best in each case.

---

587. The average duration of human gestation, when calculated from the onset of the last period, is
    A. 36 weeks
    B. 38 weeks
    C. 40 weeks
    D. 42 weeks
    E. 44 weeks

588. In measuring fundal height, the measurement should be taken
    A. from the top of the symphysis pubis in a straight line, to the top of the fundus
    B. from the ischial spines to the symphysis pubis
    C. over the bulge of the fundus
    D. diagonally, from the symphysis pubis to the top of the fundus

589. To determine the lie of the fetus within the uterus, Leopold maneuvers are performed during the midtrimester. How many Leopold maneuvers are there?
    A. 2
    B. 3
    C. 4
    D. 5
    E. 6

590. The umbilical cord normally contains
    A. two arteries and two veins
    B. two arteries and one vein
    C. one artery and two veins
    D. one vein and one artery

Explanatory Answers

491. B. The lesion described is characteristic of the primary syphilis chancre. The lesions associated with granuloma inguinale are papulonodules, which ulcerate and produce malodorous discharge. Condylomatous lesions are more "wart-like," while chancroid lesions are tender with a foul discharge. Herpes lesions are vesicular first, and then ulcerative. (Ref. 49, p. 138ff)

492. C. The FTA-ABS is a fluorescent test that detects the antibodies found in response to the causative agent *T. pallidum*. It is specific and has no false positive results, as do the RPR and VDRL. The spirochete *T. pallidum* cannot be cultured. The CRP is a seldom-used test that increases in response to many inflammatory reactions. (Ref. 49, p. 141ff)

493. D. Signs and symptoms are most suggestive of trichomonas. *Chlamydia* is not typically associated with a discharge. The discharge of *Candida* is usually white and "cheesy." *Gardnerella* is associated with a thick, grayish white, watery discharge of a "fishy" odor and "clue" cells. (Ref. 49, p. 161ff)

494. E. "Clue cells" are vaginal squamous epithelial cells with the small, pleomorphic, gram-negative coccobacilli of *Gardnerella* adhering to their surfaces. (Ref. 49, p. 162)

495. B. While many tuboovarian abscesses can be medically managed, a rupture of the abscess is a complication not to be missed. If a patient's condition worsens and rupture is suspected, surgery is essential. (Ref. 49, pp. 190–191)

496. B. High numbers of pregnancies and the use of oral contraceptions for greater than five years are thought to decrease a woman's risk of developing ovarian cancer by removing the stimulation of FSH-LH on the ovary. (Ref. 49, pp. 207–208)

497. D. In polycystic ovary syndrome, the FSH level is increased and there is unopposed estrogen stimulation of the endometria, resulting in higher risk of endometrial hyperplasia or adenocarcinoma. (Ref. 49, pp. 210–211)

498. A. The upper outer quadrant is the major site of breast cancer development. (Ref. 49, p. 222)

499. D. The best time to examine breasts is after menstruation and its accompanying fluid loss. Examination during other times is difficult, as breast engorgement develops during the latter half of the cycle. (Ref. 49, pp. 222–224)

500. C. After an initial baseline mammogram for those over 35 years old, mammograms should be done every 1 to 2 years for those ages 40 to 49, and annually over 50. (Ref. 49, p. 224)

501. C. Prior to colposcopy, many women underwent cold-knife conization for an abnormal Pap, a procedure not without hazard. There is no real correlation between the degree of dysplasia and its progression to carcinoma, so merely observing or repeating the Pap smear does not provide adequate patient evaluation. (Refs. 49, pp. 237–238; 50, pp. 496–498)

502. B. In culdocentesis, to reach the peritoneal cavity, the needle needs to be inserted into the posterior fornix. (Ref. 49, p. 240)

503. D. Cyanosis and softening of the cervix is Goodell's sign. McDonald's sign is present when the cervix may be flexed upon the corpus. Hegar's sign is softening of the isthmus of the uterus transversely. A fingertip softening of the cervical isthmus is Ladin's sign. (Refs. 48, p. 164; 49, pp. 261–262)

504. A. Cyanosis and softening of the cervix is Goodell's sign. McDonald's sign is present when the cervix may be flexed upon the corpus. Hegar's sign is softening of the isthmus of the uterus transversely. A fingertip softening of the cervical isthmus is Ladin's sign. (Refs. 48, p. 164; 49, pp. 261–262)

505. C. Cyanosis and softening of the cervix is Goodell's sign. McDonald's sign is present when the cervix may be flexed upon the corpus. Hegar's sign is softening of the isthmus of the uterus transversely. A fingertip softening of the cervical isthmus is Ladin's sign. (Refs. 48, p. 164; 49, pp. 261–262)

506. B. Cyanosis and softening of the cervix is Goodell's sign. McDonald's sign is present when the cervix may be flexed upon the corpus. Hegar's sign is softening of the isthmus of the uterus transversely. A fingertip softening of the cervical isthmus is Ladin's sign. (Refs. 48, p. 164; 49, pp. 261–262)

507. A. During pregnancy, the level of thyroid binding globulin increases and binds to the increased T4 associated with pregnancy. The free T4 remains normal. The elevated TB results in additional binding sites and the T3RU is decreased. (Ref. 49, p. 273)

508. E. While cardiac contractions of the fetal heart begin at about the 28th day, they are not detectable until day 44. (Ref. 49, p. 286)

509. B. Nagele's rule uses the date of the last day of the LMP + 7 days – 3 months. The same date can be reached by adding 280 days to the first day of the LMP, or adding 9 months and 7 days to the LMP. (Ref. 49, p. 314)

510. E. The fundal measurement correlates well with gestational development from weeks 16 through 34. Measurements below the tenth percentile at any week are suspicious for IUGR, requiring further evaluation. (Ref. 49, pp. 314–315)

511. B. In false labor, the cervix will typically dilate to 3 cm. Active labor begins after 3 cm of dilatation and gradual effacement. (Ref. 49, p. 322)

512. C. The second stage of labor varies in time from 0 to 45 minutes, depending on the parity of the patient. The third stage of labor is the time from the delivery of the infant to the delivery of the placenta. The term "fourth stage of labor" is used by some older physicians to refer to the first hour after the delivery. (Ref. 49, p. 325)

513. D. Whatever scale is used, the ischial spines represent the zero station. Here the fetal presenting part is considered "engaged." (Ref. 49, p. 325)

514. E. Given IV, Demerol rapidly leaves the fetal circulation after peaking in about six minutes, yet provides good analgesia for the mother. Meperidine can cause depressed respiratory function in the infant. Phenergan or Vistaril can be used in combination with Demerol. (Ref. 49, pp. 336–339)

515. E. The pain pathways from the perineum travel through the pudendal nerve to S2, S3, and S4. (Ref. 49, pp. 336–339)

516. D. The technique described is that of a pudendal block, as the pudendal nerve is blocked. A caudal block is placed through the sacral hiatus, an epidural at L2, L3, or L4. In a paracervical block, anesthetic is placed in the vaginal fornices. (Ref. 49, pp. 336–339)

517. C. A first-degree laceration involves only the surface epithelium. Superficial and deep tissues, but not the rectal sphincter, are involved in a second-degree laceration. If the rectal sphincter is also involved, a third-degree laceration is present. A fourth-degree laceration also involves rectal mucosa. (Ref. 49, p. 343)

518. B. A first-degree laceration involves only the surface epithelium. Superficial and deep tissues, but not the rectal sphincter, are involved in a second-degree laceration. If the rectal sphincter is also involved, a third-degree laceration is present. A fourth-degree laceration also involves rectal mucosa. (Ref. 49, p. 343)

519. D. The Apgar score is based on a one-minute and five-minute evaluation of a newborn's appearance, pulse, grimace, activity or tone, and respiration. (Ref. 49, pp. 346–347)

520. B. The Apgar score is based on giving each of five variables a score of 0, 1, or 2. (Ref. 49, pp. 346–347)

521. A. Prior to 32 weeks gestation, the head circumference is greater than the abdominal circumference; from 32 to 36 weeks they are about equal; and after 36 weeks, the abdominal circumference becomes the larger of the two. (Ref. 49, p. 385)

522. B. A threatened abortion occurs when there is bleeding and/or cramping in the first 20 weeks of pregnancy in a patient whose membranes are intact and cervix closed. An inevitable abortion also occurs in the first 20 weeks, and is associated with bleeding, cramping, dilated cervix, and/or membrane rupture, but no passage of tissue. Once tissue is passed, the abortion is incomplete (if not all passed) or complete. If the products of conception are retained for eight weeks after fetal death, the abortion is missed. (Ref. 49, pp. 391–393)

523. C. A threatened abortion occurs when there is bleeding and/or cramping in the first 20 weeks of pregnancy in a patient whose membranes are intact and cervix closed. An inevitable abortion also occurs in the first 20 weeks, and is associated with bleeding, cramping, dilated cervix, and/ or membrane rupture, but no passage of tissue. Once tissue is passed, the abortion is incomplete (if not all passed) or complete. If the products of conception are retained for eight weeks after fetal death, the abortion is missed. (Ref. 49, pp. 391–393)

524. A. A threatened abortion occurs when there is bleeding and/or cramping in the first 20 weeks of pregnancy in a patient whose membranes are intact and cervix closed. An inevitable abortion also occurs in the first 20 weeks, and is associated with bleeding, cramping, dilated cervix, and/or membrane rupture, but no passage of tissue. Once tissue is passed, the abortion is incomplete (if not all passed) or complete. If the products of conception are retained for eight weeks after fetal death, the abortion is missed. (Ref. 49, pp. 391–393)

525. D. It is felt that the effects of cigarette smoking, resulting in decreased weight of the infant, head circumference, and body length, has its greatest influence during the last four months of pregnancy. This is related to the decreased oxygenation due to carboxyhemoglobin, as well as the nicotine effect on uterine blood flow. (Ref. 49, pp. 404–405)

526. B. Vaginal colonization by group B *Streptococcus* ranges as high as 30%. It can lead to severe maternal postpartum infection, and cervical Gram stain may not be diagnostic. (Ref. 49, p. 414)

527. D. Abruptio placenta is associated with vaginal bleeding, a tense uterus, absent fetal heart tones, and shock. Maternal blood loss must be assessed along with fetal distress, and a C-section may be the treatment of choice. Placenta previa usually is associated with painless vaginal bleeding. (Ref. 49, p. 473ff)

528. E. The major cause of perinatal death in patients with placenta previa is prematurity. Beyond 37 weeks, prolonging the pregnancy will be of no added benefit to the fetus. (Ref. 49, p. 473ff)

529. B. The diagnosis of preeclampsia is defined as hypertension with edema and/or proteinuria after 20 weeks of pregnancy. Convulsions in a preeclamptic patient change the diagnosis to eclampsia. (Ref. 49, pp. 475–476)

530. A. Magnesium sulfate, IM or IV, is the drug of choice for the treatment of PIH in an attempt to stabilize the patient prior to delivery. Calcium gluconate is the antagonist for magnesium poisoning. Hydralazine can be used, in addition, to lower the blood pressure and reduce the risk of a CVA. (Ref. 49, p. 479)

531. A. Only Rho (D) negative mothers are at risk of becoming sensitized by the D antigen if present in the fetus. Those with known high antibody titers or with previous Rho (D) positive infants or unknown Rh type miscarriages or abortions may be candidates for Rho (D) immune globulin. (Ref. 49, pp. 481–482)

532. A. The normal baseline FHR is 120 to 160 bpm. Bradycardia is classified as less than 100, and tachycardia at greater than 160. Baseline FHR represents the heart rate at periods of no uterine contraction. (Ref. 49, p. 489)

533. B. The early deceleration or head compression pattern is characterized by smooth decelerations at the same time as the contractions; it is of no clinical significance. An ominous sign of fetal distress is the late deceleration or uteroplacental insufficiency pattern, in which the deceleration begins after and persists longer than the contraction. The cord compression pattern is of variable onset in relation to the contraction and can have a V-, W-, or U-shape, but its rise and fall is always abrupt. A fetal anemia pattern has a rolling baseline. (Ref. 49, p. 490ff)

534. A. The early deceleration or head compression pattern is characterized by smooth decelerations at the same time as the contractions; it is of no clinical significance. An ominous sign of fetal distress is the late deceleration or uteroplacental insufficiency pattern, in which the deceleration begins after and persists longer than the contraction. The cord compression pattern is of variable onset in relation to the contraction and can have a V-, W-, or U-shape, but its rise and fall is always abrupt. A fetal anemia pattern has a rolling baseline. (Ref. 49, p. 490ff)

535. D. Only ritodrine hydrochloride (Yutopar) is FDA-approved as a tocolytic agent, and even it has side-effects of hypotension, tachycardia, and pulmonary edema. (Ref. 49, pp. 501–502)

536. A. Both group B streptococci and *N. gonorrhoeae* are organisms that can result in fetal death secondary to infection due to premature rupture of the membranes. (Ref. 49, p. 503)

537. C. A premature fetus is one which is delivered before 38 weeks gestation. (Ref. 49, p. 504)

538. D. A complete breech is when the legs are flexed at the hips and one or both knees are also flexed. An incomplete breech can be single or double footling, and occurs when one or both hips are unflexed and one or both feet or knees are below the breech. In the frank breech position, the hips are flexed and knees extended with legs along the head. (Ref. 49, pp. 508–509)

539. D. Most occiput posterior presentations rotate during labor to occiput anterior, the easiest to deliver. While both brow and face presentations may need cesarean sections to decrease fetal problems, it is the shoulder presentation, or transverse lie, that may result in maternal death. (Ref. 49, p. 513ff)

540. E. In placenta accreta, the placenta is attached to the myometrium. If it actually invades the myometrium, it is called placenta increta. If the placenta has penetrated through the myometrium to the peritoneal surface of the uterus, it is called placenta percreta. Abruptio placenta is present if there is separation of a normally implanted placenta prior to delivery of an infant. In placenta abruptio, the placenta is implanted close to or over the os. (Ref. 49, pp. 472–475, 526–527)

541. C. In placenta accreta, the placenta is attached to the myometrium. If it actually invades the myometrium, it is called placenta increta. If the placenta has penetrated through the myometrium to the peritoneal surface of the uterus, it is called placenta percreta. Abruptio placenta is present if there is separation of a normally implanted placenta prior to delivery of an infant. In placenta abruptio, the placenta is implanted close to or over the os. (Ref. 49, pp. 472–475, 526–527)

542. E. In placenta accreta, the placenta is attached to the myometrium. If it actually invades the myometrium, it is called placenta increta. If the placenta has penetrated through the myometrium to the peritoneal surface of the uterus, it is called placenta percreta. Abruptio placenta is present if there is separation of a normally implanted placenta prior to delivery of an infant. In placenta abruptio, the placenta is implanted close to or over the os. (Ref. 49, pp. 472–475, 526–527)

543. D. Paget's disease must be considered in cases of nipple and areolar erosion, or weeping eczematoid lesions. In such cases, mammography and biopsies of the effected areas are indicated. (Ref. 50, p. 485)

544. D.   If the muscular support of the vaginal canal is damaged by stretching of childbirth, marked descent of the anterior vaginal wall and base of the bladder may occur, resulting in a cystocele. If the urethra is involved, a cystourethrocele may exist. A rectocele is suspected if the posterior vaginal wall bulges forward. (Ref. 50, pp. 401–402)

545. D.   Iron supplements are recommended for all pregnant and lactating women due to the increased demand for iron by the fetus. Calcium should usually be increased later in pregnancy and during lactation. Vitamin B_{12} may be indicated for vegetarian patients or those with megaloblastic anemias. (Ref. 48, pp. 173–174)

546. B.   While a laparoscopy and hysteroscopy might be helpful diagnostic studies in a patient with known pelvic disease or a negative D&C, a D&C should be done first in a woman with abnormal uterine bleeding. Dilatation and evacuation is an extension of the D&C, performed in abortions. (Refs. 48, p. 822ff; 49, p. 243ff)

547. A.   During menopause, the estrogen levels fall and eventually menses cease as the endometrium is no longer stimulated. FSH and LH rise to try to stimulate remaining follicles. Increased ovarian testosterone, along with decreased estrogen, can lead to mild hirsutism. (Refs. 48, p. 960ff; 49, p. 552ff)

548. A.   Most spontaneous abortions result from an abnormality with the fetus, frequently a chromosomal defect such as trisomies, monosomies, or polypoidy. While infection, diabetes, and uterine dysfunction can result in spontaneous abortions, they are less frequent causes. An incomplete cervix does not retain a fetus at 14 to 28 weeks, secondary to cervical effacement and dilatation. (Refs. 48, p. 255ff; 49, p. 391ff)

549. C.   The average amount of blood lost during menses is 25 to 60 mL. The hemoglobin begins to fall if the blood loss is 60 to 80 mL. (Refs. 48, p. 114; 49, p. 50)

550. E.   Hypermenorrhea refers to heavy or prolonged bleeding, with menorrhagia being a more specific term for heavy bleeding. Polymenorrhea means frequent periods, while amenorrhea means absent periods, and bleeding between periods is metrorrhagia. Oligomenorrhea is used to describe infrequent periods, while hypomenorrhea refers to scanty periods. (Ref. 49, p. 51)

551. C. Hypermenorrhea refers to heavy or prolonged bleeding, with menorrhagia being a more specific term for heavy bleeding. Polymenorrhea means frequent periods, while amenorrhea means absent periods, and bleeding between periods is metrorrhagia. Oligomenorrhea is used to describe infrequent periods, while hypomenorrhea refers to scanty periods. (Ref. 49, p. 51)

552. B. Hypermenorrhea refers to heavy or prolonged bleeding, with menorrhagia being a more specific term for heavy bleeding. Polymenorrhea means frequent periods, while amenorrhea means absent periods, and bleeding between periods is metrorrhagia. Oligomenorrhea is used to describe infrequent periods, while hypomenorrhea refers to scanty periods. (Ref. 49, p. 51)

553. A. Hypermenorrhea refers to heavy or prolonged bleeding, with menorrhagia being a more specific term for heavy bleeding. Polymenorrhea means frequent periods, while amenorrhea means absent periods, and bleeding between periods is metrorrhagia. Oligomenorrhea is used to describe infrequent periods, while hypomenorrhea refers to scanty periods. (Ref. 49, p. 51)

554. C. KOH can be used to highlight the hyphae and buds associated with *Candida* by eliminating debris. It is also useful with *Gardnerella,* as its addition "releases" the characteristic fishy odor. (Ref. 49, pp. 161–162)

555. B. Both *Gardnerella* and trichomonas can be successfully treated with metronidazole. *Candida* requires use of several antifungal vaginal creams (miconazole nitrate, clotrimazole, terconazole) and *Chlamydia* is treated with antibiotic regimens. (Ref. 49, p. 160ff)

556. E. All of the agents listed can cause acute inflammation of the cervix. (Ref. 49, p. 178)

557. E. Secondary dysmenorrhea is associated in the visible pelvic pathology, while primary dysmenorrhea is painful menstruation without visible pelvic pathology. (Ref. 50, pp. 177–183)

558. A. The etiology of cervical cancer remains unknown; but certain factors, such as sexual intercourse at an early age, multiple partners, and high parity are associated with a high-risk for its development. Some also feel that being of lower socioeconomic status also increases risk. (Ref. 49, pp. 181, 183)

559. A. Differentiating acute pelvic inflammatory disease from a tuboovarian abscess is essential in patient evaluation. The presentation may be identical, save for the mass. (Ref. 49, pp. 187–189)

560. E. Endometriosis, the presence of endometrial tissue in an ectopic location, is a common cause of pelvic pain. Many symptoms and signs are found in association with it, and may vary with the age of the patient and the ectopic location of the endometrium. (Ref. 49, pp. 193–194)

561. E. While all of the drugs listed can be used in treating endometriosis, danazol (Danoerine) is popular at present. The drug has a maculizing effect in a female fetus, and barrier contraception is recommended during its use. It is also costly and produces side-effects in many patients. (Ref. 49, p. 195)

562. B. A variant of polycystic ovary disease, Stein-Levanthal syndrome results from chronic anovulation. In addition to anovulation, there is usually oligomenorrhea, infertility, obesity, and hirsutism. (Ref. 49, p. 210)

563. A. Early menarche and late menopause are both risk factors for the development of breast cancer, as are obesity and a diet high in fat. Previous cancer in one breast predisposes the woman to developing breast cancer in the other breast. Increased parity leading to decreased risk, and nulliparity to increased risk, are no longer held as true by some authorities. (Ref. 49, pp. 221–222)

564. C. Endocervical cells are best found by the squamocolumnar junction scraping and endocervical swab. (Refs. 49, p. 237; 50, p. 496)

565. A. Culdocentesis can aid in the diagnosis of intraabdominal problems such as ectopic pregnancy, and tuboovarian abscesses. It is useful in following ovarian carcinoma patients. Abnormal Pap smears suggest cervical disease and colposcopy is the next diagnostic test of choice. (Refs. 49, pp. 240–244; 50, p. 40)

566. B. The pregnancy can be jeopardized if endometrial biopsies or hysteroscopies are performed. Culdocentesis may be useful in diagnosing ectopic pregnancy. (Ref. 49, p. 239ff)

567. B. A positive diagnosis of pregnancy can be made only if the fetus is detected, either by detecting its movements or heartbeats. Ultrasonography can detect fetal development by the sixth week. A positive pregnancy gives a probable, but not positive, diagnosis of pregnancy, as false positives do occur. (Ref. 49, p. 314)

568. A. All of the first three calculations estimate the date of confinement. The EDC is an estimate only accurate to within three weeks. (Ref. 49, p. 314)

569. C. The paracervical block will partially reduce the uterine contraction pain, and a regional block, such as epidural or caudal, will almost completely eliminate the pain. Risks are involved with regional blocks; however, and paracervical blocks are contraindicated in cases of fetal compromise. (Ref. 49, pp. 338–339)

570. E. All of the choices listed are potential risks, with hypotension being so severe as to result in cardiorespiratory arrest. (Ref. 49, pp. 338–339)

571. E. All of the choices listed are potential fetal risks. Maternal risks include infection and hemorrhage. (Ref. 49, p. 358)

572. A. The OCT and nipple stimulation tests are based in the fetal reaction to oxytocin, given in the OCT and stimulated by the nipple stimulation test. The NST merely records fetal heart rate over time. The L/S (lecithin/sphingomyelin) ratio, done by way of amniocentesis, is used to assess pulmonary maturity of the fetus. (Ref. 49, pp. 359–361)

573. E. While all of the conditions listed are potential causes of ectopic pregnancy, PID is the most common cause of ectopic tubal pregnancy. (Ref. 49, pp. 394–395)

574. A. Pain, amenorrhea, and vaginal bleeding are the "classic triad" of symptoms of ectopic pregnancy. Other symptoms and signs include fainting with straining at stool, syncope, shoulder pain, shock, and sanguineous nonclotting blood in the cul-de-sac. (Ref. 49, p. 395)

575. E. The symptoms of abdominal pain, nausea, and weakness in a patient who has missed a normal menses is suggestive of ectopic pregnancy. The feyer also makes it necessary to include PID, appendicitis, and tuboovarian abscess in her differential. (Ref. 49, p. 395)

576. E. All of the choices are potential causes for this woman's symptoms. Many patients with ectopic pregnancy present with only moderate symptoms. The right tube is involved more than the left. The absence of fever rules out PID, appendicitis, tuboovarian abscess, and septic abortion. (Ref. 49, p. 395)

577. D. Live vaccines should be avoided. (Ref. 49, p. 407)

578. E. All of the choices listed should cause the clinician to consider diabetes as a problem for this patient. Almost one-third of pregnant diabetics have hydramnios, and large babies and stillbirths have a high correlation to diabetes. Diabetes is suspect in any patient with monilial infections, pregnant or not. (Ref. 49, p. 451ff)

579. A. ^{131}I is contraindicated in pregnancy, but surgical and medical methods may be used. As Tapazole can cause scalp lesions in the infants of mothers treated with it, PTU is the preferred medical treatment. (Ref. 49, pp. 338–339)

580. E. An incompetent cervix can result from congenital, functional, or traumatic reasons. Any uterine malformation may be associated with a congenitally shortened cervix. Cervical conization, D&Cs, and forceps delivery all can result in excessive stretching or laceration of the cervix. (Ref. 49, p. 466)

581. E. Cerclage can salvage 80% of pregnancies where an incompetent cervix is a problem. It should only be used early, before any threatened abortion symptoms or labor is detected. (Ref. 49, pp. 369ff, 467)

582. B. The early deceleration or head compression pattern is characterized by smooth decelerations at the same time as the contractions; it is of no clinical significance. An ominous sign of fetal distress is the late deceleration or uteroplacental insufficiency pattern in which the deceleration begins after and persists longer than the contraction. The cord compression pattern is of variable onset in relation to the contraction, and can have a V-, W-, or U-shape, but its rise and fall is always abrupt. A fetal anemia pattern has a rolling baseline. (Ref. 49, p. 490ff)

583. A. While a variable baseline on a fetal monitor may indicate fetal compromise, as in hypoxia or prematurity, it may only indicate a sleeping fetus. Sedative medications may give a similar pattern. (Ref. 49, p. 493)

584. B. Caput formation and fetal head molding in an occiput anterior presentation may be an indication of fetal head elongation with the head not being engaged. C-section should be considered. (Ref. 49, p. 513)

585. E. Tace and Parlodel are used routinely to suppress lactation, as are estrogens like diethystilbesterol and ethynyl estradiol. Estrogen increase may increase the risk of thromboembolism during the puerperium. Parlodel has some unpleasant side-effects such as nausea, constipation, headache, and dizziness. (Ref. 48, pp. 243–244)

586. D. Even with low-dose pills, patients with a history of previous vascular disease such as stroke, arteriosclerosis, thrombophlebitis, and thromboembolism should not receive oral contraceptives. Diabetes, heart or liver diseases, hypertension, and breast or endometrial cancer are also contraindications. (Ref. 49, p. 574)

587. C. Normally, human pregnancy lasts 280 days, or 40 weeks, nine calendar or ten lunar months. (Ref. 48, p. 167)

588. A. The height of the fundus should be measured in a straight line over the fundus, from the top of the symphysis pubis to the top of the fundus. It should not be measured over the bulge of the fundus, as is commonly done. (Ref. 49, pp. 58–59)

589. C. There are four Leopold maneuvers. The first locates the fetal part in the fundus; the second locates the fetal back. The third maneuver locates which pole of the fetus is presently in the inlet. The fourth maneuver locates the side of cephalic prominence. (Ref. 49, pp. 59–61)

590. B. The normal cord has two arteries carrying blood from the embryo to the chorionic villi, and one umbilical vein returning blood to the embryo. A cord with one vein and one artery occurs in about 1/500 deliveries; about one-third of these infants have structural defects. (Ref. 48, pp. 143–144)

13 Health Promotion

DIRECTIONS (Questions 591–611): Each of the questions or incomplete statements below is followed by four or five suggested answers or completions. Select the **one** that is best in each case.

591. The **MOST** important modifiable cause of death is
    A. physical inactivity
    B. smoking
    C. hypertension
    D. obesity
    E. elevated blood cholesterol

592. In past decades, premature death was largely caused by infectious disease. Today it is largely a result of lifestyle-related diseases. Which of the following lifestyle diseases is the leading cause of death in the United States?
    A. Cancer
    B. Stroke
    C. Hypertension
    D. Coronary artery disease
    E. Accidents

593. The **MOST** common cancer in American men is cancer of the
    A. prostate
    B. lung
    C. stomach
    D. colon and rectum
    E. pancreas

594. The leading cause of premature cancer mortality in women is cancer of the
    A. lung
    B. colon and rectum
    C. breast
    D. cervix
    E. ovary

595. Dietary fiber is useful in the treatment and prevention of all of the following disorders **EXCEPT**
    A. glucose intolerance
    B. obesity
    C. hyperlipidemia
    D. diverticular disease
    E. gastric cancer

596. The leading contributor of deaths from cancer in the United States is cancer of the
    A. bladder
    B. colon and rectum
    C. lung
    D. breast
    E. pancreas

597. Prevention of disease before it occurs by controlling risk factors and by specific preventive services is
    A. primary prevention
    B. wellness model
    C. secondary prevention
    D. health risk analysis
    E. tertiary prevention

598. Which one of the following groups has made no documented changes in high-risk behavior in response to the human immunodeficiency virus epidemic?
A. Homosexual men
B. Bisexual men
C. Intravenous drug users
D. Adolescents
E. Heterosexual populations in high-risk areas

599. Recommended groups for counseling and testing for human immunodeficiency virus (HIV) infection include
A. people with a history of blood transfusions between 1978 and 1985
B. women whose past or present sexual partners were HIV-infected, bisexual, or intravenous drug users
C. persons with a history of multiple sexual partners
D. persons seeking treatment for sexually transmitted disease
E. all of the above

600. The **MOST** effective smoking cessation technique is
A. behavior therapy
B. a combination of strategies
C. nicotine gum
D. physician counseling
E. hypnosis

601. The process of analyzing those aspects of a given patient's medical history, physical examination, laboratory findings, and lifestyle that tend to increase or decrease the likelihood of that individual experiencing various causes of morbidity and mortality is
A. primary intervention
B. behavior modification
C. health risk appraisal
D. secondary intervention
E. wellness model

602. Which one of the following statements about breast cancer is **IN-CORRECT?**
   A. Advances in treatment have caused a dramatic decline in the age-adjusted mortality rate over the past ten years
   B. Breast cancer has been the leading cause of premature cancer mortality in women
   C. Breast cancer accounts for approximately one in four newly diagnosed cancers in women
   D. The number of breast cancer cases is expected to rise substantially over the next 40 years
   E. The three screening tests usually considered for breast cancer are clinical examination of the breast, x-ray mammography, and breast self-examination

603. Which one of the following statements about the health conse-quences of smoking is **INCORRECT?**
   A. Smoking is the most important modifiable cause of death in the United States
   B. Smoking accounts for one out of every six deaths in the United States
   C. Lung cancer has replaced breast cancer as the chief cause of cancer death in women
   D. Smoking is more common among persons of high socioeconomic status
   E. Over three-fourths of smokers begin smoking as teenagers

604. Which of the following paired types of prevention is **INCOR-RECTLY** matched?
   A. Specific preventive services—Primary prevention
   B. Prevention of disability in chronic disease—Tertiary prevention
   C. Health promotion—Primary prevention
   D. Early detection and treatment of symptomatic disease—Secondary prevention
   E. Detection of asymptomatic disease by testing/screening—Primary prevention

605. Once disease is clinically apparent, treatment aimed at restoring the patient to his or her predisease state of health is called
   A. primary prevention
   B. wellness model
   C. secondary prevention
   D. health risk analysis
   E. tertiary prevention

606. Rationale supporting PA involvement in health promotion includes all of the following **EXCEPT**
   A. the leading causes of premature death are preventable
   B. it only takes a few minutes during the PA's interaction with patients to discuss their risks and propose solutions
   C. patients entrust their health to the PA and accept his/her authority in health matters
   D. it generates more practice income through offering these services
   E. even a few minutes devoted to discussing risks and how to change lifestyles can have a demonstrable effect

607. In emphasizing the primary prevention of coronary artery disease (CAD), which of the following would **NOT** be included?
   A. Periodic screening for high blood pressure and high serum cholesterol
   B. Electrocardiogram
   C. Risk appraisal of dietary fat and cholesterol intake
   D. Risk appraisal of physical activity
   E. Risk appraisal of tobacco use

608. For **MOST** healthy persons, maximum cardiovascular fitness can be achieved by a program of vigorous aerobic exercise for
   A. 60 minutes, 2 to 4 times per week, during which a pulse rate of about $(220 - age) \times 70\%$ is reached and maintained
   B. 15 to 45 minutes, 2 to 4 times per week, during which a pulse rate of about $(220 - age) \times 70\%$ is reached and maintained
   C. 15 to 45 minutes every day, during which a pulse rate of about $(220 - age) \times 70\%$ is reached and maintained
   D. 60 minutes, 2 to 4 times per week, during which a pulse rate of about $(220 - age) \times 85\%$ is reached and maintained
   E. 15 to 45 minutes, 2 to 4 times per week, during which a pulse rate of about $(220 - age) \times 85\%$ is reached and maintained

609. The aim, in chronic diseases where disease cannot be reversed (eg, cystic fibrosis; diabetes mellitus), to optimize the quality of health by minimizing complications and preventing further progression of the disease is called
   A. primary prevention
   B. wellness model
   C. secondary prevention
   D. health risk analysis
   E. tertiary prevention

610. Which of the following statements about motor vehicle injuries is **FALSE?**
   A. Motor vehicle crashes are the leading cause of death in persons 5 to 24 years of age
   B. Because they drive less than younger persons, persons over 60 years of age have a decreased risk of motor vehicle crashes
   C. Almost half of all Americans do not use seat belts
   D. About half of fatally injured drivers are legally intoxicated with ethanol
   E. Proper use of seat belts can reduce risk of motor vehicle injury and mortality by about half

611. Which one of the following statements about acquired immunodeficiency syndrome (AIDS) is **INCORRECT?**
   A. AIDS is the only major disease in the United States in which mortality is increasing
   B. AIDS is the leading cause of death in intravenous drug users
   C. AIDS is the leading cause of death in patients with hemophilia
   D. Within ten years of human immunodeficiency virus infection, about half of persons develop AIDS
   E. AZT (azidothymidine, zidovudine) has been shown to reduce mortality in persons with AIDS

---

612. The U.S. Preventive Services Task Force guidelines on dietary counseling recommend which of the following interventions for the general population?
    1. Reduction of total fat intake to less than 30% of total calories
    2. Reduction of dietary cholesterol to less than 300 mg per day
    3. Reduction of saturated fat consumption to less than 10% of total calories
    4. Reduction of dietary sodium from 4 to 6 grams per day

613. Clinicians should provide all patients with information on the role of physical activity in disease prevention and assist in selecting an appropriate type of exercise. Which of the following statements is/are **TRUE** in reference to designing an exercise program for a patient?
    1. Medical limitations need to be considered
    2. The patient should be encouraged to set at least one specific exercise goal; the target heart rate should be only a small increment above baseline status
    3. Activity characteristics that both improve health and enhance compliance need to be considered
    4. Beginners should emphasize vigorous, rather than regular, exercise

614. Which of the following forms of cancer is/are **MOST** closely associated epidemiologically with nutritional risk factors?
    1. Colon
    2. Breast
    3. Prostate
    4. Lung

615. Conservative weightloss regimens reported as having the lowest failure rates involving persons with mild to moderate obesity include
  1. behavior therapy
  2. surgery
  3. exercise programs
  4. insertion of a gastric balloon

616. Physical inactivity has been associated with a number of debilitating medical conditions in the United States, including
  1. coronary artery disease
  2. hypertension
  3. noninsulin-dependent diabetes mellitus
  4. osteoporosis

617. Weight loss reduces an individual's risk for which of the following major chronic diseases?
  1. Diabetes mellitus
  2. Hypertension
  3. Coronary artery disease
  4. Cirrhosis

618. Condoms have been shown to decrease the rate of transmission of which of the following?
  1. Human immunodeficiency virus
  2. Gonorrhea
  3. *Chlamydia*
  4. Herpes

Directions Summarized				
A	**B**	**C**	**D**	**E**
1,2,3	1,3	2,4	4	All are
only	only	only	only	correct

619. According to the U.S. Preventive Services Task Force guidelines, which of the following patients is/are candidates for intensive counseling about the dietary management of hyperlipidemia?

1. A 45-year-old man with an average serum cholesterol of 260 mg per dL, and no other cardiac risk factors
2. A 50-year-old woman with an average serum cholesterol of 235 mg per dL, a high-density lipoprotein cholesterol less than 35 mg per dL, and no other cardiac risk factors
3. A 60-year-old man with an average serum cholesterol of 195 mg per dL, who is a smoker, but has no other cardiac risk factors
4. A 55-year-old man with an average serum cholesterol of 195 mg per dL, who is a smoker, is hypertensive, and has a positive family history of premature coronary artery disease

620. Warning signs of overexertion for those undertaking exercise conditioning include

1. a heart rate over 120 beats per minute, two minutes following the cessation of exercise
2. extreme fatigue ten minutes after an exercise routine
3. persistent tiredness and trouble sleeping during the day following exercise
4. pressure in the chest

621. Which of the following statements regarding exercise is/are **TRUE?**

1. Studies have shown that men who are physically active on a regular basis have a lower overall mortality than those who are physically inactive
2. Physically inactive persons are twice as likely to develop coronary artery disease as are persons who engage in regular physical activity
3. Weightbearing physical activity may reduce bone loss in postmenopausal women
4. Incidence of clinically confirmed psychiatric disorders can be reduced through exercise

622. Key tools of health promotion include
1. health education
2. disease prevention
3. health protection
4. coercive behavior change methods

623. The definition of health education implies which of the following assumptions?
1. The principal goal of health education is health enhancing behavior
2. Voluntary participation is an essential element of health education; coercion is not education
3. Health education requires multiple approaches; there are no "magic bullet" methods
4. Health education should be carefully planned using behavioral and educational diagnostic techniques

624. At what level can a PA provide health and prevent disease?
1. He/she can work directly with patients
2. He/she can intervene at work to encourage changes in health-related policy, resources, and programs
3. In the community, he/she can serve as a health advocate
4. He/she can join the political process and influence legislation that affects health

625. Health promotion and disease prevention have become national issues in response to the realization that
1. the power of traditional curative medicine is limited
2. lifestyle and health are related
3. the cost of health care is rising sharply
4. people can be prompted to voluntarily change their lifestyle practices through health education and related organizational (such as workplace), political, or economic measures

Explanatory Answers

591. B.   Smoking accounts for one out of every six deaths in the United States. It is the most important modifiable cause of death. (Ref. 51, p. 289)

592. D.   Coronary artery disease is the leading cause of death in the United States, accounting for about 1.5 million myocardial infarctions and over 520,000 deaths each year. (Ref. 51, p. 297)

593. A.   Prostate cancer is the most common cancer in American men, and has the third highest cancer mortality rate. (Ref. 51, p. 63)

594. C.   Breast cancer is the leading contributor to premature cancer mortality in women. (Ref. 51, p. 39)

595. E.   Increased intake of dietary fiber improves gastric motility. Certain types of dietary fiber may also be helpful in the treatment of glucose intolerance, weight reduction, and the control of lipid disorders. A high-fiber diet may be effective in reducing intracolonic pressure and preventing diverticular disease. (Ref. 51, p. 307)

596. C.   Cancer of the lung is the leading cause of death from cancer in the United States. (Ref. 51, p. 67)

597. A.   Preventing disease before it occurs by controlling risk factors and by specific preventive services (immunizations, nutrition, genetic counseling, environmental control measures, etc.) is called primary prevention. (Ref. 54, pp. 44, 154)

598. D.   Evidence from recent surveys indicates that changes in high-risk behavior is not occurring dramatically in certain population groups, such as adolescents. (Ref. 51, p. 334)

599. E.   Counseling and testing for HIV should be offered to persons seeking treatment for sexually transmitted diseases, persons with a history of prostitution or multiple sexual partners, homosexuals and bisexual men, past or present IV drug users, and women whose past or present sexual partners were HIV-infected. Bisexual or IV drug users, persons with long residence or birth in an area with a high prevalence of HIV infection, and persons with a history of transfusions between 1978 and 1985 also should be tested. (Ref. 51, p. 143)

600. B. The most effective techniques are those meeting more than one modality (eg, physician advice; self-help materials), those involving physicians and nonphysicians, and those that provide the greatest number of motivational messages for the longest period of time. (Ref. 51, p. 291)

601. C. Health risk appraisal is the process of analyzing those aspects of a given patient's medical history, physical examination, laboratory findings, and lifestyle that tend to increase or decrease the likehood of that individual experiencing various causes of morbidity or mortality. (Ref. 54, p. 50)

602. A. The age-adjusted mortality rate from breast cancer has been almost unchanged over the past ten years. (Ref. 51, p. 39)

603. D. Cigarette smoking is more common among blacks and persons of low socioeconomic status. (Ref. 51, p. 289)

604. E. The detection of asymptomatic disease by testing/screening (eg, vision; hearing; stool for occult blood) is primary prevention. (Ref. 54, p. 45)

605. C. Secondary prevention includes activities directed at the early detection and treatment of existing disease to interrupt the progression of the disease process or to minimize disability. (Ref. 54, pp. 44, 154)

606. D. Generating more practice income is not a valid reason for PA involvement in health promotion. (Ref. 54, p. 49)

607. B. Clinicians should emphasize the primary prevention of CAD by periodically screening for high blood pressure and high serum cholesterol and by routinely investigating behavioral risk factors for CAD such as tobacco use, dietary fat and cholesterol intake, and inadequate physical activity. Secondary prevention of CAD (screening) by performing routine electrocardiography to screen asymptomatic persons is not recommended as an effective strategy to reduce the risk of CAD. (Ref. 51, p. 6)

608. B. For most healthy persons, maximum cardiovascular fitness can be achieved by a program of vigorous aerobic exercise for 15 to 45 minutes, two to four times per week, during which a pulse rate of about (220 − age) × 70% is reached and maintained. (Ref. 51, p. 301)

609. E. Tertiary prevention includes activities directed toward the alleviation of disability resulting from disease. Efforts to restore function and productivity of the patient represent one of many sophisticated activities of this level of care. (Ref. 54, pp. 44, 154)

610. B. The risk of motor vehicle crashes is also increased for persons over age 60; but elderly motorists account for only 20% of fatal crashes, primarily because they drive less than younger persons. (Ref. 51, p. 315)

611. E. In a study performed before the licensure of AZT, only half of patients survived one year beyond diagnosis; the five-year survival rate was only 15%. (Ref. 51, p. 139)

612. A. Adolescents and adults, in particular, should be given dietary guidance in how to reduce total fat intake to less than 30% of total calories and dietary cholesterol to less than 300 mg per day. Saturated fat consumption should be reduced to less than 10% of total calories. (Ref. 51, p. 309)

613. A. Beginners should emphasize regular, rather than vigorous, exercise. (Ref. 51, p. 301)

614. A. Cancer of the colon, breast, and prostate, the three forms of cancer most closely associated epidemiologically with nutritional risk factors, together cause over 130,000 deaths annually. (Ref. 51, p. 305)

615. B. Although a variety of weight-reducing regimens are available, many have only short-term efficacy and fail to result in long-term weight loss. The lowest failure rates have been reported for conservative weight loss regimens such as behavior therapy, nutrition education, and exercise programs, primarily involving persons with mild to moderate obesity. (Ref. 51, p. 112)

616. E. Physical inactivity has been associated with coronary artery disease, noninsulin-dependent diabetes mellitus, and osteoporosis. (Ref. 51, p. 297)

617. A. Weight loss reduces an individual's risk for major chronic diseases such as diabetes, hypertension, and coronary artery disease. (Ref. 51, p. 113)

618. E. Condoms have been shown in the laboratory to prevent transmission of *C. trachomatis, Herpes simplex* virus, trichmonas, cytomegalovirus, HIV, and gonorrhea. (Ref. 51, p. 333)

619. B. All adults with high blood cholesterol (at or above 240 mg per dL) and those persons with borderline high cholesterol (200 to 239 mg per dL) who have known coronary artery disease or two or more cardiac risk factors should receive information about the meaning of the results, intensive dietary counseling, and follow-up evaluation. (Ref. 51, p. 17)

620. E. Awareness of the warning signs of overexertion is a must for those undertaking exercise conditioning. Warning signs include a heart rate over 120 beats per minute two minutes following the cessation of exercise, extensive fatigue, and persistent tiredness and trouble sleeping during the day following exercise. A more serious sign would be pressure in the chest. (Ref. 52, p. 34)

621. A. A commonly mentioned benefit of regular exercise is improved affect (positive mood, reduced depression, lowered anxiety). It is known that physically active persons report higher levels of self-esteem, perhaps in response to improved personal appearance and self-image. However, no well-designed studies have shown that the incidence of clinically confirmed psychiatric disorders can be reduced through exercise. (Ref. 51, p. 297)

622. A. Key tools of health promotion are disease prevention, health protection, and health education. (Ref. 54, p. 43)

623. E. The definition of health education implies certain important assumptions including the following. (1) Health education requires multiple approaches; there are no "magic bullet" methods. (2) Health education should be carefully planned, using behavioral and educational diagnostic techniques. (3) The principle goal of health education is health-enhancing behavior. (4) Voluntary participation is an essential element of health education; coercion is not education. (Ref. 54, p. 44)

624. E. PAs can provide health and prevent disease at four levels. They can work directly with their patients. They can intervene where they work to encourage changes in health-related policy, resources, and programs. In the community, they can take several roles as health advocates. Last, they can join the political process and influence legislation and regulation that affect health. (Ref. 53, p. 87)

625. E.   The realization that the power of tradition curative medicine is limited, that lifestyle and health are related, and that the cost of health care is rising sharply have made health promotion and disease prevention national issues. (Ref. 53, p. 96)

14 Neurology and Endocrinology

DIRECTIONS (Questions 626–660): Each of the questions or incomplete statements below is followed by four or five suggested answers or completions. Select the **one** that is best in each case.

626. A 68-year-old man presents with a history of intermittent ptosis and diplopia. Examination demonstrates fatigable proximal arm muscles and bilateral medial rectus muscle weakness with a left lid ptosis. The **MOST** likely diagnosis is
   A. brainstem stroke
   B. polymyositis
   C. myasthenia gravis
   D. multiple sclerosis
   E. muscular dystrophy

627. Reversible causes of dementia include all of the following **EXCEPT**
   A. Alzheimer's disease
   B. thyroid disease
   C. vitamin B_{12} deficiency
   D. intracranial mass lesions
   E. depression

628. Cluster headaches are associated with all of the following **EXCEPT**
   A. males are affected more than females
   B. tearing of the affected eye
   C. headaches lasting for days at a time
   D. nasal blockage or discharge
   E. ergotamine preparations can suppress attacks

629. After a comatose patient has been stabilized, which of the following steps should be taken **FIRST**?
   A. Order a CT scan of the head
   B. Obtain an EKG
   C. Place a nasogastric tube
   D. Insert a Foley catheter
   E. Start IV and give 50% dextrose

630. Bacterial meningitis
   A. in pediatric patients is **MOST** often caused by *S. pneumoniae*
   B. is associated with normal glucose on CSF examination
   C. produces a mononuclear cell predominance in CSF
   D. usually presents with headache and fever
   E. always presents with stiff neck

631. Computed tomography may assist in the detection of all of the following neurologic disorders **EXCEPT**
   A. mass lesions
   B. demyelinating disease
   C. cerebral hemorrhage
   D. hydrocephalus
   E. cerebral atrophy

632. Which of the following statements about carpal tunnel syndrome is **FALSE**?
   A. The median nerve is entrapped at the wrist
   B. Symptoms include numbness and tingling of the thumb, index, and middle fingers, and half of the ring finger
   C. A positive Tinel's sign is elicited by sudden flexion of the wrist
   D. Predisposing factors include obesity, pregnancy, and occupational uses of the wrist, such as typing
   E. Treatment is effected by surgically decompressing the nerve

633. In the newly diagnosed Parkinson's disease patient, your initial approach to treating a mild tremor would be
   A. low-dose anticholinergic agent
   B. bromocriptine
   C. levodopa
   D. amantadine
   E. a combination of anticholinergic agent and levodopa

634. Dose-related side-effects of phenytoin therapy include all **EXCEPT**
   A. ataxia
   B. nystagmus
   C. dysarthria
   D. osteomalacia

635. Pharmacologic and nonpharmacologic measures employed in the prophylaxis of migraine headaches include all of the following **EXCEPT**
   A. beta-adrenergic blocking agents
   B. ergotamine
   C. tricyclic antidepressants
   D. calcium channel blockers
   E. biofeedback and relaxation exercises

636. Your patient is a 20-year-old woman recently diagnosed with epilepsy. She is anxious about the effect her disease will have on her life. Which of the following patient education points is **INCORRECT**?
   A. Most states require a one-year seizure-free period before granting driving privileges
   B. There are few areas of employment which preclude the hiring of someone with a seizure disorder
   C. There is no need for concern about passing the disease on to her offspring
   D. Since alcohol may stimulate seizure activity, abstinence may be necessary

637. In patients over the age of 50, the **MOST** common cause of new onset of seizures is
A. brain tumors
B. cerebrovascular disease
C. metabolic disorders
D. trauma
E. congenital malformations

638. A left homonymous hemianopsia indicates a lesion located at the
A. optic chiasm
B. right optic nerve
C. left optic tract
D. right optic tract

639. All of the following may be prominent clinical features of Parkinson's disease **EXCEPT**
A. slowness of movement
B. fixed facial expression
C. tremor that is most pronounced at rest
D. dementia in the late stages of the disease
E. ataxic gait

640. The single **MOST** important piece of information you can obtain in evaluating the patient with dizziness is
A. a description of what the patient means by "dizziness"
B. whether or not there is an associated loss of hearing
C. precipitating factors
D. a drug history
E. a precise account of the timing of the dizziness

641. Clinical manifestations of thoracic outlet syndrome include all of the following **EXCEPT**
A. increased deep tendon reflexes in the affected limb
B. sensory loss most pronounced in the fourth and fifth fingers
C. color changes in the hand
D. weakness of the ulnar portion of the hand
E. pain in the arm in certain positions

642. You are evaluating an elderly gentleman for dementia. Initially, the test which will be **MOST** useful to you is
A. EEG
B. lumbar puncture
C. brain biopsy
D. thyroid function tests
E. arteriography

643. Features which characterize trigeminal neuralgia include all of the following **EXCEPT**
A. patients may be at risk for suicide because of the severity of pain
B. surgery provides the usual initial approach to treatment
C. anticonvulsants have proven somewhat effective in managing pain
D. attacks may be triggered by minor contact with a trigger zone

644. In educating your patient with chronic low back pain, you should mention all of the following **EXCEPT**
A. use a footrest when standing for long periods
B. bend your knees and use your leg muscles when lifting
C. sleeping flat on the back will help prevent recurrence
D. get regular exercise, such as walking or swimming
E. when sitting, try to keep knees higher than hips

645. A 32-year-old construction worker has suffered a disc herniation involving the S1 nerve root. You would expect this patient to exhibit which of the following signs or symptoms?
A. Diminished ankle reflex
B. Great toe pain
C. Diminished or absent knee jerk
D. Quadriceps weakness
E. Numbness of the medial thigh and leg

646. Reported precipitants of migraine headaches include all of the following **EXCEPT**
A. emotional stress
B. foods cured with nitrates
C. oral contraceptives
D. beta-blockers
E. alcohol

647. The patient with a true dementia will
  A. usually have a history of psychopathology
  B. often answer "I don't know" to questions
  C. retain good attention and concentration
  D. show rapid progression of symptoms
  E. have a greater loss for recent, rather than remote, events

648. A 41-year-old man presents with a single thyroid nodule, enlarged lymph nodes, and a remote history of neck irradiation. The **MOST** likely diagnosis is
  A. thyroiditis
  B. thyroid carcinoma
  C. benign thyroid nodule
  D. follicular adenoma
  E. multinodular goiter

649. Clinical features of hypothyroidism include all of the following **EXCEPT**
  A. carpal tunnel syndrome may be a presenting symptom
  B. fatigue and cold intolerance may be early symptoms
  C. weakness and heat intolerance may be early symptoms
  D. deep tendon reflexes may show a delayed relaxation phase
  E. severe disease may result in variable degrees of heart block

650. Symptoms of hyperglycemia include all of the following **EXCEPT**
  A. diaphoresis
  B. polydipsia
  C. weight loss
  D. blurred vision
  E. polyuria

651. A 19-year-old woman takes 20 units of NPH insulin and seven units of regular insulin in the morning. Fasting blood sugars have been 100 to 110 mg/dL. Late in the afternoon, she often notes mild irritability, sometimes accompanied by headache. To relieve this, you could recommend
  A. beginning a mid-afternoon exercise program
  B. adding a mid-afternoon snack
  C. increasing her regular insulin dosage in the morning
  D. adding five units of regular insulin before dinner
  E. taking aspirin as needed for headaches

652. Drug causes of gynecomastia include all of the following **EXCEPT**
- **A.** digoxin
- **B.** spironolactone
- **C.** cimetidine
- **D.** alcohol
- **E.** beta-blockers

653. Diagnostic tests that may be useful in the evaluation of Cushing's syndrome include all of the following **EXCEPT**
- **A.** dexamethasone suppression test
- **B.** plasma ACTH
- **C.** abdominal CT scan
- **D.** urinary 17-ketosteroids
- **E.** serum potassium

654. All of the following hormones are produced by the anterior pituitary **EXCEPT**
- **A.** ACTH
- **B.** LH
- **C.** TSH
- **D.** ADH
- **E.** FSH

655. Diabetes insipidus is due to a deficiency in
- **A.** insulin
- **B.** vasopressin
- **C.** adrenocorticotropic hormone
- **D.** prolactin
- **E.** aldosterone

656. The **MOST** likely cause of hypercalcemia in the asymptomatic patient is
- **A.** hyperparathyroidism
- **B.** malignancy
- **C.** ingestion of calcium
- **D.** hyperthyroidism
- **E.** Addison's disease

657. The diagnosis of primary hypothyroidism can be made by demonstration of
   A. a low T4 and a low TSH
   B. a low T4 and a high TSH
   C. a small increase in TSH in response to TRH administration
   D. a low TSH and a low thyroid-binding globulin

658. Adrenal crisis is characterized by all of the following **EXCEPT** it
   A. may complicate the course of Cushing's syndrome
   B. is a potentially lethal complication of Addison's disease
   C. may be stimulated by the presence of infection
   D. is treated by infusion of cortisol, sodium, and water

659. Osteomalacia is caused by a deficiency in
   A. vitamin A
   B. vitamin B_{12}
   C. vitamin C
   D. vitamin D
   E. vitamin E

660. Risk factors for development of osteoporosis include all of the following **EXCEPT**
   A. lack of exercise
   B. early menopause
   C. excessive alcohol consumption
   D. female gender
   E. black race

DIRECTIONS (Questions 661–675): For each of the questions or incomplete statements below, **one or more** of the answers or completions given are correct. Select:

A   if only **1, 2,** and **3** are correct,
B   if only **1** and **3** are correct,
C   if only **2** and **4** are correct,
D   if only **4** is correct,
E   if **all** are correct.

661. Characteristics of type I diabetes mellitus include
   1. ketosis prone
   2. insulin resistance common
   3. juvenile onset
   4. often obese

662. Which of the following statements regarding diet should you include in counseling your newly diagnosed type II diabetic patient?
   1. Diet should be high in complex carbohydrates
   2. High fiber intake will improve glucose tolerance
   3. Diet composition is less important than achieving ideal body weight
   4. Diet exchange systems are necessary in the absence of insulin dependence

663. Complications of diabetes mellitus include
   1. cataracts
   2. renal insufficiency
   3. myocardial infarction
   4. gastroparesis

664. A 47-year-old asymptomatic man presents for follow-up of recently diagnosed mild diastolic hypertension, for which he is being treated with hydrochlorothiazide, 50 mg daily. Routine laboratory workup reveals a serum calcium of 10.4 mg/dL. Appropriate initial action would include
   1. serum parathyroid hormone level
   2. CT scan of the neck
   3. IVP
   4. discontinuation of hydrochlorothiazide and rechecking of calcium in two months

	Directions Summarized			
A	**B**	**C**	**D**	**E**
1,2,3	1,3	2,4	4	All are
only	only	only	only	correct

665. Which of the following patient education points would you want to make to your patient on chronic glucocorticosteroid therapy?
    1. Steroids may be taken with food without impairing absorption
    2. Contact health care provider if subjected to unusual stress or illness
    3. Take medication in the morning to prevent HPA suppression
    4. Do not stop taking medication abruptly

666. Acromegaly
    1. is usually caused by pituitary adenoma
    2. is associated with an increase in adrenocorticotropic hormone
    3. causes facial disfiguring, fatigue, and increased sweating
    4. is generally treated medically

667. Drugs used in the management of thyrotoxicosis include
    1. propilthiouracil (PTU)
    2. beta-blocking agents
    3. potassium iodide (SSKI)
    4. radioactive iodine (^{131}I)

668. Which of the following is/are recognized side-effects of long-term glucocorticosteroid therapy?
    1. Glucose intolerance
    2. Osteoporosis
    3. Psychosis
    4. Cataracts

669. Conditions associated with hirsutism include which of the following?
1. Cushing's syndrome
2. Hyperthyroidism
3. Phenytoin therapy
4. Thiazide diuretic therapy

670. A 28-year-old woman presents with a one-month history of tiredness, nervousness, and palpitations. She tells you that she read an article about hypoglycemia and thinks this may account for her symptoms. Things you should be aware of with regard to hypoglycemia include which of the following?
1. The oral glucose tolerance test should be used in all patients suspected of being hypoglycemic
2. Patients who think they are hypoglycemic are often found to be suffering from underlying emotional problems
3. Everyone with a blood sugar of 35 to 45 mg/dL will experience symptoms of hypoglycemia
4. Fasting hypoglycemias are more serious than the postprandial variety

671. Masked hyperthyroidism in the elderly is characterized by
1. unexplained heart failure
2. atrial fibrillation
3. new onset of a psychiatric disorder
4. tremor

672. Which of the following is/are **TRUE** statement(s) regarding glucose intolerance and pregnancy?
1. Fetal hyperglycemia can result in excessive fetal growth
2. All pregnant women should be screened for glucose intolerance
3. Diabetic women who become pregnant may require adjustments in insulin dosage
4. All pregnant patients with glucose intolerance should be treated with insulin

		Directions Summarized		
A	**B**	**C**	**D**	**E**
1,2,3	1,3	2,4	4	All are
only	only	only	only	correct

673. Prominent symptoms of a carotid TIA include
 1. paresthesias
 2. paresis
 3. loss of vision in one eye
 4. vertigo

674. A 30-year-old executive presents with recent onset of bilateral bandlike headaches, which worsen as the day progresses. The **MOST** useful tool in your initial diagnostic workup of this patient is
 1. a complete history
 2. CT of the head
 3. neurologic examination
 4. cervical spine x-rays

675. Clinical features of Bell's palsy include which of the following?
 1. Involvement of the peripheral seventh cranial nerve
 2. Involvement of a central, supranuclear facial nerve lesion
 3. Upper and lower parts of the face are involved
 4. Lower face only is involved

Explanatory Answers

626. C. Myasthenia gravis has a peak incidence in older adults. It is characterized by weakness and fatigability, usually beginning in the extraocular muscles with ptosis and diplopia. Repetitive movements of the arm muscles may cause weakness. Diplopia is uncommon in muscular dystrophies, as both eyes are affected symmetrically. Fatigability is the feature which distinguishes myasthenia from the other disorders. (Ref. 55, pp. 760–761)

627. A. Alzheimer's disease is a progressive, irreversible disorder, causing slow decline in cognitive function and resulting in a terminal vegetative state. Pseudodementia may be the presenting feature in depressive illnesses. Treatment of metabolic and endocrine disorders as well as intracranial tumors may reverse their associated dementias. (Ref. 55, pp. 686–689)

628. C. Cluster headaches tend to occur in bouts over several weeks to months. Most attacks last only minutes to several hours. The pain typically centers around one eye, leading to tearing and nasal symptoms ipsilaterally. Treatment is often anticipatory, using ergotamine at bedtime to suppress symptoms. (Ref. 2, p. 2505)

629. E. Initially, the management of a comatose patient centers on stabilization. While waiting for blood chemistries, dextrose should be administered via IV. Coma due to hypoglycemia will be reversed by this intervention without risk even to the patient who may be suffering from diabetic ketoacidosis. (Ref. 2, pp. 2531–2532)

630. D. In children, the most common agent of infection is *H. influenzae*. Patients often present with fever, headache, and alterations in consciousness. About 80% will complain of stiff neck. CSF examination reveals a fall in glucose and >50% neutrophils. (Ref. 55, pp. 568–569)

631. B. CT is helpful in detecting structural abnormalities, but may not have the necessary resolution to detect arteriovenous malformations or demyelination. (Ref. 55, p. 672)

632. C. Carpal tunnel syndrome is the entrapment of the median nerve as it passes through the flexor retinaculum, which causes pain and paresthesias to the involved fingers. Symptoms occur more at night and may result in sensory loss and weakness. Predisposing factors include occupational overuse, pregnancy, myxedema, and RA. Light tap over the wrist causes paresthesias (Tinel's sign). The most effective treatment is surgical release. (Ref. 55, p. 754)

633. A. If a mild tremor is well tolerated, no medication need be started; but if symptoms are distressing, a low dose of anticholinergic, such as Artane, will generally be well-tolerated and effective. This avoids the more serious side-effects of the other anti-Parkinson drugs. (Ref. 57, pp. 753–754)

634. D. Osteomalacia is related to the duration of exposure to phenytoin, rather than to the dosage. Ataxia, nystagmus, dysarthria, and blurred vision are all dose-related side-effects. (Ref. 57, p. 743)

635. B. Ergotamine is used to treat an acute attack of migraine and is most effective when taken at the first sign of headache. Verapamil appears to be effective in preventing headaches. Tricyclics decrease the frequency of migraine, especially in patients with depressive symptoms. Propranolol is effective in reducing the severity and frequency of attacks for about two-thirds of patients. (Ref. 57, pp. 749–750)

636. C. Epilepsy is hereditary and between 25% and 33% of patients have a family history of the disease. State driving laws vary, but most have the one-year seizure-free law. Only pilots and people requiring a chauffeur's license are unable to work with seizure disorder. Alcohol, coffee, and tobacco may all stimulate seizure activity. (Ref. 57, p. 744)

637. B. (Ref. 58, p. 1971)

638. C. Fibers from the right temporal and left nasal fields travel together in the right optic tract and radiation. Interruption of these fibers will result in loss of vision in those fields. (Ref. 58, p. 1982)

639. E. The gait of Parkinson's disease is a stooped, festinating one, with difficulty in starting and stopping. (Ref. 58, pp. 2065–2066)

640. A. Differentiating between true vertigo, faintness, postural instability, and a feeling of lightheadedness will guide the direction of further questioning. (Ref. 57, p. 723)

641. A. Deep tendon reflexes remain normal in thoracic outlet syndrome. (Ref. 57, p. 727)

642. D. A search for treatable causes of dementia should begin with noninvasive blood studies, a good history, and physical examination. (Ref. 57, pp. 737–738)

643. B. Surgery is reserved for those cases which are refractory to medical treatment. Drugs commonly used to manage pain in these patients include carbamazepine, phenytoin, and baclofen. (Ref. 57, pp. 762–763)

644. C. When sleeping on the back, a pillow should be placed under the knees to help flatten the lower back against the mattress. (Ref. 57, p. 656)

645. A. The areas affected by the S1 root includes the lateral ankle and foot, posterior thigh and calf, and buttock. (Ref. 57, p. 652)

646. D. Beta-blockers tend to reduce the frequency and severity of migraine headaches, and are often employed in their pharmacologic treatment. (Ref. 57, p. 749)

647. E. Demented patients will try hard to compensate for their cognitive loss, but will suffer from poor concentration and a gradual, slow loss of function. Many people suffering from dementias have no past psychiatric history. Recent memory is affected to a much greater extent than remote memory. (Ref. 59, p. 97)

648. B. The above presentation would be consistent with carcinoma about 30% of the time. Hoarseness would be another likely symptom. (Ref. 55, p. 464)

649. C. Weakness and heat intolerance are symptoms of hyperthyroidism. (Ref. 55, p. 462)

650. A. Diaphoresis is a symptom of hypoglycemia. (Ref. 55, p. 498)

651. B. The symptoms she experiences indicate low blood sugar late in the afternoon. A snack at mid-afternoon would prevent this trough. Increasing or adding to existing insulin regimens would only exacerbate the problem. (Ref. 57, pp. 478–480)

652. E.   (Ref. 57, pp. 472–473)

653. E.   The dexamethasone suppression test determines the presence of Cushing's syndrome. Elevation of plasma ACTH or the presence of adrenal mass or hyperplasia on abdominal CT help to pinpoint the cause, as does abnormality of urinary excretion of 17-KS. Serum potassium should not be affected. (Ref. 58, pp. 1720–1724)

654. D.   Antidiuretic hormone is produced by the posterior pituitary. (Ref. 58, p. 1655)

655. B.   Diabetes insipidus is a disorder in which large quantities of dilute fluid are lost in the urine, and is due to either the failure of the kidney to respond to vasopressin release or failure of the pituitary gland to release the hormone in spite of physiologic stimuli. (Ref. 59, pp. 1684–1686)

656. A.   About 60% of those with asymptomatic hypercalcemia have primary hyperparathyroidism. (Ref. 57, p. 461)

657. B.   (Ref. 57, pp. 491–492)

658. A.   Acute adrenocortical insufficiency intensified by sepsis or other forms of stress, characterizes adrenal crisis. Patients with Addison's disease should be aware of those settings in which they should increase their hormone dosage. They should also be aware of the consequences of abrupt withdrawal of hormone replacement. Treatment is aimed at replacement of sodium and water deficits, as well as rapid increase in circulating glucocorticoid. (Ref. 58, p. 1732)

659. D.   (Ref. 58, p. 1931)

660. E.   Black women have a lower rate of osteoporosis than white women and appear to have a higher bone mineral content and reduced bone resorption. (Ref. 58, p. 1922)

661. B.   Peak age of onset of type I diabetes mellitus is 11 to 13. Patients tend to be of normal weight, require insulin for control, and are prone to ketosis. Insulin resistance is uncommon. (Ref. 55, p. 497)

662. A.   Special exchange diets are no longer recommended for type II diabetics. Weight loss for those above ideal body weight is essential. High fiber and high carbohydrate diets have proven useful in improving glycemic control. (Ref. 57, p. 476)

663. E. (Ref. 57, pp. 480–481)

664. D. Thiazide diuretics are known to cause elevations in serum calcium. Before proceeding with expensive workup for this borderline elevation, a trial discontinuation of the suspected offending agent seems appropriate. Repetition of the lab test is also reasonable given the rate of false elevations reported. (Ref. 55, pp. 521–522)

665. E. (Ref. 57, pp. 497–499)

666. B. Acromegaly occurs as a result of growth hormone excess associated with pituitary tumors in the lateral wings of the sella. Enlargement and coarsening of facial features, hands, and feet occurs, and the basal metabolic rate increases, causing sweating and fatigue. Treatment of choice remains transsphenoidal ablation of the tumor. (Ref. 58, pp. 1662–1664)

667. E. (Ref. 57, pp. 486–488)

668. E. Other effects include myopathies, fat redistribution, and, infrequently, peptic ulceration. (Ref. 57, pp. 494–495)

669. B. (Ref. 57, pp. 468–470)

670. C. Hypoglycemia is diagnosed when symptoms occur with a documented low blood sugar (<45 mg/dL). Some individuals are asymptomatic with such blood sugars. Fasting hypoglycemias are caused by autonomous insulin secretion, overuse of exogenous insulin, or defects in glucoregulatory mechanisms. People with emotional problems often seek a medical explanation to account for their symptoms. (Ref. 57, pp. 464–467)

671. A. Hyperthyroidism in the elderly may present atypically in about 25% of cases. Masked hyperthyroidism refers to the disease which presents in ways that suggest other diseases, ie, heart failure, tachyarrhythmias, psychiatric disorders, and myopathies. Tremor is a typical finding in hyperthyroidism. (Ref. 59, pp. 277–278)

672. A. Complications of fetal hyperglycemia include high birth weight, leading to increased caesarean sections, birth trauma, and neonatal respiratory problems. Because of the risk of morbidity and mortality to the fetus, all pregnant women should be screened by the 24th to 28th week of gestation. Diabetics may require a lowering of insulin dosage during the first trimester and an increase during the second trimester. Many glucose intolerant pregnant women can be managed by dietary restriction alone. (Ref. 57, p. 481)

673. A. Vertigo occurs commonly in vertebrobasilar TIAs. (Ref. 59, p. 259)

674. B. The quality, location, and course of a headache, as well as associated symptoms, will give many clues in diagnosing the cause of headaches. A thorough physical examination with attention to vital signs, eyes, ears, sinuses and cranial arteries, mouth, and neck is also warranted, and may reveal a source. A neurologic examination is essential because a focal finding may indicate an intracranial lesion. Radiologic studies are reserved for patients with findings from the history and physical examination which warrant their use. (Ref. 57, pp. 717–719)

675. B. Bell's palsy is an acute facial paralysis affecting the peripheral seventh nerve and presenting with unilateral drooping eyelid, face, and mouth. A central lesion affects only the lower face muscles. (Ref. 57, p. 760)

15 Emergency Medicine

DIRECTIONS (Questions 676–720): Each of the questions or incomplete statements below is followed by four or five suggested answers or completions. Select the one that is best in each case.

676. Immediate treatment of a patient who presents with a severe, systemic reaction to a bee sting should be
    A. aerosol aqueous epinephrine 1:1000
    B. subcutaneous aqueous epinephrine 1:1000
    C. subcutaneous epinephrine 1:10,000
    D. an alpha-agonist agents (eg, pseudoephedrine)

677. Corneal abrasion may best be managed with all of the following **EXCEPT**
    A. saline irrigation of the eye
    B. topical antibiotics
    C. mydriatics to relax the ciliary muscle
    D. topical anesthetics

678. Removal of a simple, foreign body of the cornea is **BEST** accomplished by using a
    A. fine-gauge needle or spud
    B. soft, cotton-tip applicator
    C. battery-operated drill with a burr tip
    D. normal saline high-pressure irrigation

679. Blunt facial trauma involving the eye which results in restricted eye movement in upward gaze, diplopia, and decreased sensation over the maxilla is **MOST** likely caused by a/an
- **A.** orbital floor "blowout" fracture
- **B.** retinal detachment
- **C.** maxillary (Le Fort 1) fracture
- **D.** periorbital hematoma

680. The electrocardiogram finding **MOST** consistent with atrial fibrillation is
- **A.** progressive prolongation of the PR interval
- **B.** a widened QRS complex with an inverted T wave
- **C.** atrial rate 250 to 350 beats per minute with a "saw-tooth" configuration
- **D.** atrial rate greater than 350; no P wave; irregularly, irregular ventricular response

681. A five-year-old child ingests an unknown quantity of aspirin. The father frantically phones the ER where you work. They live 30 minutes away by car. At this time the child is alert. You advise the father to
- **A.** do nothing until they reach the ER
- **B.** induce vomiting
- **C.** have the child drink high-glucose beverages
- **D.** not worry, he only needs to be sure there is adequate fluid intake over the next 24 hours

682. The initial pharmacologic treatment of a patient with the presumptive diagnosis of pulmonary embolism is
- **A.** epinephrine 1:1000
- **B.** heparin
- **C.** morphine
- **D.** aminophylline

683. In the immediate treatment of a patient with status epilepticus, you would administer which of the following medications?
- **A.** Phenytoin (Dilantin)
- **B.** Diazepam (Valium)
- **C.** Phenobarbital
- **D.** Primidone (Mysoline)

684. While working in the emergency room, you are monitoring a patient with blunt head trauma, and you note that the patient has developed hypertension. Your treatment of this problem would be
  A. elevation of the patient's feet
  B. reduction of intracranial pressure
  C. administering an antihypertensive medication
  D. emergency burr holes

685. In monitoring the response of a patient under treatment for an acute asthmatic attack, the laboratory test/method considered **MOST** useful is
  A. arterial blood gases
  B. chest x-ray
  C. electrocardiography
  D. spirometry

686. In evaluation of a patient who has overdosed on a sedative-hypnotic drug, you find that the pupillary light reflex is present and responsive to light. Which of the following sedative/hypnotics would **NOT** produce this type of pupillary response?
  A. Chlordiazepoxide (Librium)
  B. Diazepam (Valium)
  C. Glutethimide (Doriden)
  D. Meprobamate (Equanil, Miltown)

687. Which treatment is **NOT** usually indicated in the immediate management of an uncomplicated myocardial infarction?
  A. Oxygen at 2 to 5 liters per minute
  B. Lidocaine intravenously
  C. Nitroglycerin
  D. Morphine sulfate intravenously

688. The **MOST** effective method in rapidly lowering increased intracranial pressure (secondary to trauma) would be
  A. corticosteroids
  B. osmotic diuretics given intravenously
  C. hyperventilation via endotracheal airway
  D. emergency burr holes

689. The procedure of choice in the evaluation of a patient with blunt trauma to the abdomen for intraabdominal bleeding is
    A. abdominal x-ray in the left-lateral decubitus position
    B. serial hemoglobin measurements
    C. percussion of the abdomen for "shifting dullness"
    D. peritoneal lavage

690. An asymmetrically enlarged pupil in an unresponsive patient (secondary to head trauma) may imply transtentorial herniation and should be treated with all of the following **EXCEPT**
    A. endotracheal intubation
    B. hyperventilation
    C. lumbar puncture
    D. diuretics

691. In the immediate treatment of carbon monoxide poisoning, you should administer oxygen at which of the following concentrations?
    A. 80%
    B. 75%
    C. 60%
    D. 100%

692. Inspiratory stridor, intercostal retractions, mild cyanosis, and a respiratory rate of 30/min in an afebrile child would **MOST** likely be caused by
    A. epiglottitis
    B. laryngotracheobronchitis
    C. upper airway obstruction
    D. bronchiolitis

693. When whole blood must be administered to a patient, without the benefit of typing, you would give
    A. O type, Rh^+
    B. AB type, Rh^-
    C. AB type, Rh^+
    D. O type, Rh^-

694. In selecting insulin for treatment of severe diabetic ketoacidosis, you would use
  A. crystalline (regular) insulin—intravenously
  B. NPH (isophane) insulin—intravenously
  C. lente (insulin zinc) insulin—intravenously
  D. protamine zinc (PZI) insulin—intravenously

695. Suspected alkali or acid burns to the eye should be managed with all of the following **EXCEPT**
  A. neutralizing solutions
  B. systemic analgesics
  C. topical anesthetics
  D. copious irrigation with an isotonic saline solution

696. Which of the following blood tests would **NOT** be indicated in a rape victim?
  A. Blood chemistry studies
  B. Serologic test for syphilis
  C. Blood typing
  D. Blood cultures

697. Physical signs of vascular compromise in a dislocation or fracture include all of the following **EXCEPT**
  A. pain
  B. pallor
  C. flaccid muscle tone
  D. pulselessness

698. Chest pain that is described as markedly worse on inspiration would be considered
  A. neurasthenic
  B. pleuritic
  C. anginal
  D. ischemic

699. The goal of therapy in treating a patient in shock should be to
  A. normalize the blood pressure
  B. optimize tissue perfusion
  C. maintain consciousness
  D. correct volume depletion

700. Which electrocardiographic findings are **MOST** consistent with a myocardial infarction?
A. Widened QRS complex, depressed ST segment, abnormal Q waves
B. Shortened PR interval, depressed ST segment, abnormal Q waves
C. Nonspecific ST-T wave changes, abnormal Q waves
D. High-voltage T waves, elevated ST segments, abnormal Q waves

701. The organ system **MOST** sensitive to lead poisoning is the
A. nervous system
B. reproductive system
C. urinary system
D. hematopoietic system

702. The **MOST** common signs/symptoms of ibuprofen (Motrin, Advil) intoxication in children include abdominal pain, vomiting, and
A. apnea
B. seizures
C. drowsiness
D. central nervous system depression

703. An acute onset of tachypnea, dyspnea, pleuritic chest pain and a grossly normal chest x-ray, and ECG is **MOST** suggestive of
A. pneumothorax
B. myocardial infarction
C. pulmonary edema
D. pulmonary embolism

704. A patient with an ice pick stab wound to the right anterior chest is brought to your facility complaining of worsening dyspnea. He appears cyanotic, and the blood pressure readings are falling steadily. Your presumptive diagnosis is
A. tension pneumothorax
B. acute pulmonary edema
C. pneumothorax
D. flail chest

705. Treatment of first-degree burns includes all of the following **EX-CEPT**
- **A.** washing the wound with bland soap
- **B.** tetanus immunization
- **C.** systemic analgesics
- **D.** prophylactic systemic antibiotics

706. The **MOST** common injury resulting from blunt trauma to the abdomen is
- **A.** splenic rupture
- **B.** pelvic fracture
- **C.** liver laceration
- **D.** ruptured bladder

707. Loss (or obliteration) of the psoas shadow on an abdominal x-ray, of a patient with blunt trauma to the abdomen, may indicate
- **A.** abscess formation
- **B.** retroperitoneal hematoma
- **C.** perforated viscus
- **D.** none of the above

708. Utilizing the "rule of nines" in the assessment of an adult patient with burns to the head, neck, chest, and abdomen would be considered what percentage?
- **A.** 36%
- **B.** 27%
- **C.** 18%
- **D.** 45%

709. The initial dose of naloxone (Narcan) administered to a comatose patient suspected of being a heroin abuser would be
- **A.** 4.0 mg IV
- **B.** 0.04 mg IV
- **C.** 0.4 mg IV
- **D.** 40 mg IV

710. An overdose of which antihypertensive medication will manifest the same signs and symptoms as an opiate overdose?
A. Clonidine (Catapres)
B. Enalopril (Vasotec)
C. Reserpine (Serpasil)
D. Hydralazine (Apresoline)

711. The preferred anatomical site for performing a lumbar puncture in an adult patient is
A. L1-L2
B. L5-S1
C. L3-L4
D. L2-L3

712. Basophilic stippling is seen in which of the following heavy metal poisonings?
A. Arsenic
B. Iron
C. Mercury
D. Lead

713. Detection of a pericardial friction rub within a few hours after the onset of symptoms of acute myocardial infarction might suggest the diagnosis of
A. cardiac tamponade
B. pericarditis
C. cardiac lipoma
D. myocarditis

714. The initial drug of choice in the treatment of a patient in the emergency room with an acute hypertensive crisis (BP 240/130 mm Hg), without abnormal neurologic findings, is
A. nitroprusside (Nitropress)
B. hydralazine (Apresoline)
C. methyldopa (Aldomet)
D. nifedipine (Procardia)

715. In the physical examination of a patient complaining of acute, colicky, abdominal pain, auscultation of the abdomen reveals intermittent peristaltic rushes that are synchronous with the pain. This is **MOST** diagnostic of

    A. gastroenteritis
    B. biliary colic
    C. small bowel obstruction
    D. subacute pancreatitis

716. Which of the following is acceptable in the initial treatment of a comatose patient?

    A. Glucose 50 g of a 50% solution intravenously
    B. Naloxone (Narcan) intravenously
    C. Thiamine 100 mg intravenously
    D. All of the above

717. A four-year-old child aspirates a peanut and is having difficulty breathing due to coughing and wheezing. On physical examination, you observe there is moderate cyanosis, supraclavicular retractions, and asymmetric breath sounds. The **BEST** course of action should be

    A. bronchoscopy
    B. laryngoscopy
    C. an incision over the cricothyroid
    D. a transverse incision over the trachea

718. A woman, late in her third trimester, presents to the emergency room with bright red vaginal bleeding with no abdominal pain. The blood clots well, and her blood pressure is 120/80 mm Hg. The **MOST** probable diagnosis is

    A. inevitable abortion
    B. placenta previa
    C. abruptio placentae
    D. incompetent cervix

719. Loss of consciousness followed by a brief, lucid interval (usually of less than 24 hours), followed by neurologic deterioration in a patient with head trauma is typical of
  A. acute subdural hematoma
  B. cerebral contusion
  C. subarachnoid hemorrhage
  D. acute epidural hematoma

720. The passenger of vehicle involved in a head-on collision is brought into the emergency room for evaluation and treatment. In addition to other PE findings, you note that the left leg is slightly adducted, internally rotated, and mildly flexed. This is **MOST** likely caused by
  A. anterior hip dislocation
  B. fracture of the acetabulum
  C. posterior hip dislocation
  D. fracture of the femoral neck

DIRECTIONS (Questions 721–742): For each of the questions or incomplete statements below, **one or more** of the answers or completions given are correct. Select:
  A if only **1, 2,** and **3** are correct,
  B if only **1** and **3** are correct,
  C if only **2** and **4** are correct,
  D if only **4** is correct,
  E if **all** are correct.

---

721. Treatment of heat stroke includes
  1. application of cool or iced water
  2. indwelling urinary catheter
  3. chlorpromazine to prevent shivering
  4. providing supplemental oxygen

722. The nephrotoxic agents that are the leading causes of acute renal failure include
  1. heavy metals
  2. radiographic contrast agents
  3. nonsteroidal antiinflammatory agents
  4. aminoglycoside antibiotics

723. An 82-year-old patient presents with significant epistaxis. Physical examination identifies the bleeding site as high on the posterior lateral wall of the right nostril. Management of this patient would include
1. anterior nasal packs bilaterally
2. hospitalization
3. arterial ligation
4. posterior nasal pack

724. A patient arrives at the emergency room with complaints of severe, excruciating pain of her entire right hand. She gives a history of spilling acid on herself while etching a stained glass window. You note small areas of localized erythema, without blistering, on the dorsum and fingertips of her right hand, which seems disproportionate to the amount of pain she is exhibiting. Your **IMMEDIATE** treatment would include
1. flushing the area copiously with water
2. hospitalizing for observation
3. applying/administering calcium gluconate regionally
4. atropine IV

725. Contraindications for nasogastric intubation (for gastric evacuation or lavage) include
1. massive facial trauma
2. ingestion of a caustic substance (eg, lye)
3. esophageal atresia
4. basilar skull fracture

726. Evaluation of a near-drowning victim includes
1. chest x-ray
2. patient temperature
3. acid–base status
4. integrity of the cervical spine

727. Characteristic indicators of opiate (narcotic) withdrawal include
1. lacrimation
2. yawning
3. rhinorrhea
4. myalgia

		Directions Summarized		
A	**B**	**C**	**D**	**E**
1,2,3	1,3	2,4	4	All are
only	only	only	only	correct

728. Common causes of upper gastrointestinal bleeding include
1. peptic ulceration
2. variceal bleeding
3. erosive gastritis
4. gastric carcinoma

729. Complications of electrical injuries include
1. muscle necrosis
2. myoglobinuria
3. cardiac arrhythmias
4. delayed hemorrhage

730. Treatment of a black widow spider bite, in an otherwise healthy adult, would appropriately include
1. administration of antivenom
2. confinement and observation of the spider for ten days
3. local application of heat
4. administration of muscle relaxant, ie, calcium gluconate

731. Management of hypovolemic shock in the multiply injured patient may include
1. type O negative blood
2. normal saline or lactated Ringer's intravenously
3. plasma substitutes
4. use of military antishock trousers (mast suit)

732. Systemic causes of hypothermia include
1. ethanol intoxication
2. hypothyroidism
3. drug intoxication
4. hypoglycemia

733. Clinical signs of a basilar skull fracture include
   1. regional ecchymosis (mastoid region)
   2. leakage of cerebrospinal fluid from ear or nose
   3. hemotympanum
   4. cranial nerve palsies

734. Objective signs of papilledema include
   1. hyperemic disk
   2. venous congestion
   3. retinal hemorrhages
   4. enlargement of blind spot

735. Ionizing radiation exposure may produce
   1. GI bleeding
   2. skin erythema
   3. sterility
   4. bone marrow injury

736. MAJOR burns, as classified by the American Burn Association, include
   1. most electrical burns
   2. most second- or third-degree burns of the hands or feet
   3. third-degree burns of 10% of adult body surface area
   4. second-degree burns of 40% of adult body surface area

737. High-risk factors for developing serious complications from a burn injury are patients with
   1. diabetes mellitus
   2. renal failure
   3. chronic pulmonary disease
   4. history of myocardial infarction

738. Which should be AVOIDED in the emergency treatment of a non-poisonous snake bite?
   1. Vigorous activity
   2. Ice pack on the bite area
   3. Immediate incision and suction of wounds
   4. Elastic bandage applied firmly around bite site

Directions Summarized				
A	**B**	**C**	**D**	**E**
1,2,3	1,3	2,4	4	All are
only	only	only	only	correct

739. Side-effects that can occur after using "crack" cocaine include
1. seizures
2. death
3. hypertension
4. hyperthermia

740. Management of a 75-year-old patient with a nose bleed coming from the posterior lateral wall of the nose includes
1. hospitalization
2. posterior nasal packing
3. bilateral anterior nasal packing
4. arterial ligation

741. A 70-year-old patient presents with cardiac arrhythmias secondary to chronic digitalis toxicity. Included in your initial treatment would be
1. potassium
2. calcium
3. lidocaine
4. DC countershock

742. Emergency treatment of acute adrenal insufficiency should include
1. intravenous infusion of 5% dextrose in normal saline
2. supplemental potassium
3. hydrocortisone (Cortisol) IV
4. sodium nitroprusside

DIRECTIONS (Questions 743–750): The group of questions below consists of lettered headings followed by a list of numbered words, phrases, or statements. For each numbered word, phrase, or statement, select the **one** lettered heading that is most closely associated with it. Each lettered heading may be selected once, more than once, or not at all.

Questions 743–746: Match the dominate breath odors associated with the poisonings listed.
- **A.** Pears
- **B.** Garlic
- **C.** Bitter almond
- **D.** Rotten eggs

743. Arsenic

744. Cyanide

745. Hydrogen sulfide

746. Chloral hydrate

Questions 747–750: Match the arrhythmia to the underlying condition.
- **A.** Myocardial infarction
- **B.** Thyrotoxicosis
- **C.** Syncopal episodes
- **D.** Pericarditis

747. Atrial fibrillation

748. Ventricular fibrillation

749. Elevated ST segments; peaked (tall) T waves

750. Sinus bradycardia

Explanatory Answers

676. B. Severe reactions must be treated promptly, as they may cause rapid systemic decompensation and death. Aerosol aqueous epinephrine is not adequate as a first-aid measure in treating systemic anaphylaxis. (Ref. 58, p. 438)

677. D. Topical anesthetics should not be given to a patient for repeated use after a corneal injury, as this may delay healing and mask further damage, leading to permanent scarring of the cornea. (Ref. 63, p. 344)

678. A. A cotton-tip applicator will generally remove too much of the epithelium, often without removing the foreign body; a burr tip is generally used for deeply embedded foreign bodies; and high-pressure irrigation of the eye is never indicated. (Ref. 63, p. 344)

679. A. Suspect a blowout fracture in any patient who has sustained blunt ocular trauma. Diplopia and restricted upward gaze occur when there is entrapment of the ocular muscle. Ocular injuries are usually associated with pure blowout fractures. (Ref. 58, p. 237)

680. D. Atrial fibrillation is the only common arrhythmia in which the ventricular rate is rapid and very irregular. In atrial fibrillation, impulses are blocked at the AV node, which causes an irregular ventricular response. (Ref. 58, p. 492)

681. B. Salicylates can be recovered from the body in substantial amounts for as long as 20 hours following accidental or intentional ingestion. (Ref. 57, pp. 952–953)

682. B. Anticoagulation is preventative rather than definitive therapy, as it reduces the rate of recurrent emboli. Heparin is the anticoagulant of choice and should be used if embolization is strongly suspected. Do not give if septic emboli is suspected. (Ref. 61, p. 193)

683. B. Diazepam is fast-acting, has a short half-life intravenously, and is lipid-soluble effective in 80% to 90% of cases of status epilepticus. Phenytoin is used as maintenance therapy and is preferred over phenobarbital because it does not cause respiratory depression and therapeutic brain drug levels are achieved rapidly. (Ref. 58, pp. 93–99)

684. B. Hypertension resulting from head trauma is a reflex response that is an attempt to maintain cerebral perfusion in the presence of raised intracranial pressure. (Ref. 58, pp. 204–205)

685. D. Forced expiratory volume, peak expiratory flow rate, vital capacity, and total lung capacity are all measured in spirometry. It is considered the single most useful method for judging severity and monitoring response. (Ref. 58, p. 531)

686. C. Glutethimide (Doriden) overdose is the only exception to the rule of pupillary sparing. Glutethimide regularly produces pupils fixed in mid-position and unreactive to light. (Ref. 58, pp. 88–89)

687. C. A goal of therapy in a patient with a myocardial infarction is to reduce ventricular filling pressures and to increase cardiac output. Nitrates will not increase cardiac output and may cause hypotension severe enough to decrease profusion to vital organs. (Ref. 59, pp. 161–162)

688. C. Hyperventilation by means of an endotracheal airway produces cerebral vasoconstriction and helps control cerebral swelling. It is considered one of the most effective methods of rapidly producing a decrease in intracranial pressure. (Ref. 58, p. 204)

689. D. Lavage fluid with a hematocrit of 1% or higher indicates significant intraperitoneal hemorrhage and suggests the need for laparotomy. (Ref. 58, pp. 260–261)

690. C. Lumbar puncture should not be done when head injury is an obvious or likely diagnosis. Abnormal results on lumbar puncture, with either bloody or xanthochromic fluid or elevated cerebrospinal fluid pressures, do not localize or define an intracranial abnormality. (Ref. 58, pp. 46, 207)

691. D. Carbon monoxide binds to hemoglobin with an affinity about 200 times greater than that of oxygen. To prevent neurologic damage, 100% oxygen should be administered by rebreathing face mask or endotracheal tube. The half-life of carboxyhemoglobin in a person breathing room air is 5 to 6 hours; in 100% oxygen, it is only one hour. (Ref. 58, p. 458)

692. C. Severe upper airway obstruction is characterized by inspiratory and expiratory stridor, ineffective inspiratory efforts characterized by suprasternal, supraclavicular, and intercostal retractions, often coupled with cyanosis. The diagnosis can be confirmed by asking the patient to speak. (Ref. 58, p. 53)

693. D. Universal donor blood is O type, Rh⁻. (Ref. 58, pp. 603–604)

694. A. An initial loading dose of regular insulin by rapid intravenous injection should be given as soon as the diagnosis of diabetic ketoacidosis is made. This loading dose permits rapid achievement of adequate therapeutic levels of insulin and avoids the one-hour delay associated with obtaining an effective insulin concentration at tissue receptor sites. (Ref. 58, pp. 563–564)

695. A. *Do not* attempt to neutralize the alkali or acid, since the heat generated by the chemical reaction may cause further injury. (Ref. 58, p. 383)

696. D. Whether the rape victim is male or female, blood chemistry studies, serologic tests for syphilis, and blood typing (to compare with the alleged assailant's type with that of the victim) are indicated. (Ref. 58, pp. 341–344)

697. C. A pale, cold, painful, pulseless limb is typical of arterial injury; however, sensory loss may be the only early indication of vascular compromise. (Ref. 58, p. 278)

698. B. The pain associated with pneumonia, pulmonary embolism, or isolated pleuritis is described as markedly worse on inspiration. The pain of pneumothorax, pneumomediastinum, ruptured esophagus, pericarditis, and, occasionally, myocardial infarction is frequently pleuritic in nature. (Ref. 58, p. 69)

699. B. Shock is a complex acute cardiovascular syndrome that results in a critical reduction of perfusion of vital tissues. There is the temptation to use vasoconstrictors to maintain adequate blood pressure, which will therefore increase coronary perfusion. However, this gain may be offset by increased myocardial oxygen demands, as well as more severe vasoconstriction in the blood vessels. (Ref. 59, p. 103)

700. D. Signs of myocardial infarction (seen in approximately 50% of patients) include high-voltage T waves, elevated ST segments, and abnormal-appearing Q waves. Note that a normal ECG does not rule out the possibility of a myocardial infarction. (Ref. 58, p. 482)

701. D. Lead induces critical derangements in the heme biosynthesis and shortens the lifespan of the erythrocytes. Even at very high blood levels, some individuals have no apparent neurologic manifestations. Lead nephropathy, or infertility, occurs only after years of prolonged exposure. (Ref. 58, p. 465)

702. C. Most exposures do not produce symptoms. When symptoms do occur, the more common are abdominal pain, vomiting, and drowsiness. The more unusual manifestations of ibuprofen intoxication include metabolic acidosis, apnea (especially in young children), seizures, and CNS depression. (Ref. 57, p. 944)

703. D. When embolization occurs, the consequences and manifestations depend on the size of the embolism and the underlying cardiorespiratory status. Obstruction of a localized portion of the pulmonary vascular tree causes local atelectasis, with resulting ventilation–perfusion abnormalities and hypoxemia. Reflex hyperventilation with resultant hypocapnia and tachycardia also occur. The ECG is usually normal except for a tachycardia. (Ref. 58, p. 537)

704. A. In tension pneumothorax, air continues to enter (but not leave) the pleural space during respiratory efforts, because the defect in the lung acts as a one-way valve, and pleural pressure becomes greater than atmospheric pressure. This usually shifts the mediastinum toward the contralateral uninvolved lung, compressing it and obstructing venous return to the heart. (Ref. 58, p. 527)

705. D. Prophylactic systemic antibiotics are usually not indicated in a first-degree burn (which, by definition, only involves the superficial epidermis). (Ref. 58, p. 413)

706. A. Even trivial trauma has been reported to cause splenic rupture. The spleen is highly vascular, but friable, and bleeds profusely when injured. (Ref. 64, pp. 585–599)

707. B. Flat plate abdominal x-ray and CT scan are definitive diagnostic studies to rule out a retroperitoneal hematoma. (Ref. 58, pp. 114–116)

708. B. Accurate measurement of the burned areas, expressed as a percentage of body surface area, should be performed in all burn patients. Head and neck, 9%; right arm, 9; left arm, 9%; front torso (chest and abdomen), 18%; back torso (upper back and buttocks), 18%; right leg, 18%; left leg, 18%; and genitalia and perineum, 1%. (Ref. 58, pp. 412–413)

709. C. Naloxone is a narcotic antagonist and should be given to all patients suspected of opiate overdose. Naloxone has a half-life of one hour. Carefully observe the patient for withdrawal symptoms caused by naloxone, as chronic heroin abusers may develop acute narcotic withdrawal syndrome when administered naloxone. (Ref. 58, p. 470)

710. A. Side-effects of clonidine include central nervous system depression with manifestations similar to opiate withdrawal. The patient will fail to respond to naloxone (Narcan). (Ref. 58, p. 470)

711. C. Lumbar puncture should enter the subarachnoid space below the level of the conus medullaris. L3-L4 is at the level of the posterior iliac crests. (Ref. 61, p. 828)

712. D. Basophilic stippling refers to fine blue granules enclosed in the cell: they usually represent reticulocytes. Basophilic stippling occurs in almost all patients with lead poisoning. (Ref. 58, p. 465)

713. B. The detection of a friction rub in a patient with the diagnosis of an MI is distinctly unusual and suggests the possibility of a preexisting heart disease or another diagnosis, ie, acute pericarditis. (Ref. 55, p. 485)

714. D. Nifedipine is a potent vasodilator that is used sublingually to lower blood pressure within minutes, and the dose can be titrated easily. Nitroprusside acts within seconds, but requires intraarterial pressure monitoring with the patient in an ICU. Hydralazine is not as rapid-acting and may cause an undesired tachycardia. With methyldopa, the onset of effect is not rapid, and it must be given slowly over 2 to 4 hours. (Ref. 58, pp. 510–512)

715. C. Peristaltic rushes have no relationship to the pain experienced with gastroenteritis, biliary colic, or subacute pancreatitis. (Ref. 58, p. 111)

716. D. If there is even a remote possibility that the coma may be due to opiate overdose or hypoglycemia, Narcan and/or 50% glucose should be administered intravenously. A patient with a severe thiamine deficiency may present in a coma. Failure to initiate prompt therapy in a patient with any of these features may result in death or irreversible brain damage. (Ref. 56, p. 120)

717. A. Foreign bodies in the lower respiratory tract are preferably managed by rigid, not flexible, bronchoscopy. (Ref. 57, pp. 374–375)

718. B. Painless hemorrhage is the cardinal sign of placenta previa. Although spotting may occur during the first and second trimesters of pregnancy, the first episode of hemorrhage usually begins at some point after the 28th week, and is characteristically described as being sudden, painless, and profuse. (Ref. 60, p. 395)

719. D. The majority of patients with epidural hematomas are unconscious when first seen, with a characteristic "lucid interval" of several minutes to hours before coma supervenes. The majority of patients with a subdural hematoma are drowsy or comatose from the moment of injury. Because the mass effect of the hemorrhage and rise in intracranial pressure may be life-threatening, it is important to make an immediate diagnosis. (Ref. 56, pp. 1962–1963)

720. C. Hip dislocations occur when the passenger's knee strikes the dashboard in a head-on collision. Most hip dislocations are posterior. Anterior dislocations are characterized by flexion, external rotation, and abduction of the leg. (Ref. 58, p. 299)

721. E. Act quickly to prevent further injury: maintain adequate ventilation, reduce body temperature promptly, reduce shivering, monitor urinary output. (Ref. 58, p. 429)

722. C. In the past, heavy metals were common inducers of acute renal failure; however, these toxins are less frequently encountered today. More recent studies suggest that aminoglycosides and radiographic contrast agents are the leading causes. There is a 10% to 20% incidence of acute renal failure in those patients receiving aminoglycoside antibiotics. Patients with underlying renal disease, particularly diabetic patients (radiographic studies are done more frequently in these groups), have a 10% to

40% frequency of acute renal failure following the introduction of radiographic contrast agents. (Ref. 56, p. 1149)

723. E.   Older patients often present the most difficult problem in nasal bleeding. Calcified arteriosclerotic vessels are often responsible for the bleeding; and because of their inelasticity and ineffective vasospasm, bleeding is usually profuse and difficult to stop. The quickest way to stop bleeding in a patient with suspected posterior epistaxis is to first place a posterior pack in the nasopharynx and then pack the nasal chamber anteriorly on both sides. Patients with posterior nasal packing must be hospitalized. (Ref. 58, pp. 351–352)

724. A.   Hydrofluoric acid is a powerful inorganic acid whose toxicity is due to its corrosiveness. The hallmark of toxicity is pain way out of proportion to the extent of injury present. Hydrofluoric acid readily penetrates intact dermis, and dissociates and releases fluoride, which will remain active until medically deactivated. (Ref. 62, p. 403)

725. E.   The patient must be able to swallow at the right time and the esophageal lumen cannot be severely narrow. Gentle pressure must be applied to insert the tube posteriorly and perpendicular to the long axis of the head. Any disruption (ie, basilar fracture; massive facial trauma) may allow the tube to enter the cranial vault. (Ref. 58, p. 806)

726. E.   Hypoxemia begins within seconds of submersion, and ineffective circulation begins about 2 to 4 minutes later; vasoconstriction will occur in the presence of metabolic acidosis; an initial chest x-ray is indicated in all near-drowning victims. (Ref. 61, p. 433)

727. E.   Opiates act on the central nervous system receptors and cause sedation, hypotension, bradycardia, hypothermia, and respiratory depression. (Ref. 58, p. 740)

728. A.   Relative incidence of upper gastrointestinal hemorrhage: peptic ulcer, 45%; esophageal varices, 20%; gastritis, 20%. Gastric carcinoma is a rare cause of upper GI bleeding. (Ref. 64, p. 479)

729. E.   Rhythm disturbances may develop, as the pathway of the electrical current may include the cardiac muscle. Myoglobinuria will occur following massive muscle destruction and also indicates acidosis. Burn injuries may appear innocuous despite extensive deep tissue destruction.

Ischemia and sloughing may not be evident for 7 to 10 days. (Ref. 58, pp. 430–431)

730. D.   Calcium gluconate intravenously is often effective in alleviating muscle spasm. Antivenom should be reserved for use in seriously ill infants and older patients, and should be preceded by horse serum sensitivity testing. There is no value in observing a spider for any length of time. (Ref. 58, p. 439)

731. E.   Hypovolemic shock may result from loss of whole blood, plasma, or fluid and electrolytes. Crystalloids (normal saline, lactated Ringer's) metabolize to bicarbonates, are readily available and relatively inexpensive, and effectively restore vascular volume for short periods. Colloids (blood, plasma substitutes) do not easily diffuse across normal capillary membranes. This property may enable these fluids to be retained longer in the intravascular space. Colloids also cause volume expansion, which prevents accumulation of pulmonary interstitial fluid that would hinder oxygen diffusion. Mast suits are useful in controlling hemorrhage for bleeding below the level of the diaphragm. (Ref. 58, pp. 31–35)

732. E.   Systemic hypothermia may follow exposure to even slightly lowered temperatures when there is preexisting altered homeostasis as a result of debility or disease. It is more likely to occur in elderly or inactive people with cardiovascular disease, myxedema, mental retardation, and alcohol abuse. (Ref. 58, pp. 422–423)

733. E.   Basilar skull fractures can occur at any point in the base of the skull, but the typical location is in the petrous portion of the temporal bone. This area is also known as the basilar sinus, and houses the seventh and eighth cranial nerves. (Ref. 62, p. 830)

734. E.   Papilledema is caused by increased intravascular pressure that is transmitted to the subarachnoid space around the optic nerves. Vascular changes are usually secondary phenomena. (Ref. 56, p. 73)

735. E.   Harm derived from radiation exposure depends on the quantity and type of radiation delivered to the body, and the site and duration of exposure. Injury to bone marrow may cause a decrease in the production of blood elements (lymphocytes are most sensitive); male sterility may be transient or permanent depending on the dose; females generally experience permanent sterility; loss of mucosa with ulceration and inflammation produce GI bleeding. (Ref. 58, pp. 431–432)

736. A. The first three choices are a summary of the American Burn Association burn severity categorization. (Ref. 58, p. 412)

737. E. Major existing medical problems in a burn patient are associated with an increased rate of serious complications even if their burns are not serious. Poor perfusion, delayed healing, and depressed immune system are all important factors. (Ref. 58, p. 414)

738. B. If at all possible, a person who has suffered a snake bite should avoid exertion. When a bite has been inflicted by a nonvenomous snake, it should be treated as a puncture wound. (Ref. 58, p. 436)

739. E. Cocaine has sympathomimetic effects manifested by initial excitement and seizures, followed by depression of the central nervous system. Inhalation of "crack" results in very high levels with peak effects occurring rapidly, usually in less than 30 minutes. The toxic dose varies widely among susceptible individuals. (Ref. 58, p. 460)

740. E. Older patients often present the most difficult problem in nasal bleeding. The source of bleeding is usually high and in the posterior part of the nose. Calcified arteriosclerotic vessels are often responsible for the bleeding, and because of their inelasticity and ineffective vasospasm, bleeding is usually profuse and difficult to stop. The quickest way to stop bleeding in a person with suspected posterior epistaxis is to first place a posterior pack in the nasopharynx and then pack the nasal chamber anteriorly on both sides. (Ref. 58, p. 352)

741. B. Serious toxic effects are those that cause rhythm and conduction disturbances in the heart. Hypokalemia will aggravate digitalis toxicity in a patient on chronic therapy. DC countershock should be avoided because it may cause serious conduction and rhythm disturbances. Use of calcium may potentiate the existing cardiac toxicity. Lidocaine is indicated for ventricular ectopic beats. (Ref. 58, p. 459)

742. B. Treatment is primarily directed toward the rapid elevation of circulation glucocorticoid and the replacement of sodium and water deficits. Hence, an intravenous infusion of 5% glucose in normal saline solution should be immediately started with a bolus IV infusion of 100 mg

Cortisol. Synthetic glucocorticoids (eg, prednisolone or dexamethasone) cause less sodium retention and should probably not be used in an acute situation. Replacement therapy for potassium (if needed) should be started when the serum potassium begins to fall after hydration and cortisol administration. Usually a patient with acute adrenal insufficiency is hypotensive and, therefore, nitroprusside is contraindicated. (Ref. 56, p. 1772)

743. B. Many agents, when absorbed and metabolized, give a charac-
744. C. teristic breath odor. A definitive diagnosis should never be
745. D. made solely by identification of a breath odor; however, in
746. A. situations where rapid identification is necessary, and there is are no laboratory services available, presumptive treatment may be lifesaving. (Ref. 58, p. 747)

747. B. Atrial fibrillation frequently occurs in pulmonary embolism,
748. A. mitral valve disease, thyrotoxicosis, acute myocardial infarc-
749. D. tion, and potassium deficiency. Acute myocardial infarction is
750. C. the most common cause of ventricular fibrillation, although patients with coronary artery disease may have VF without preceding infarction, and VF often accompanies drowning and electrocution, and digitalis, quinidine, or procainamide toxicity. (Refs. 55, pp. 458–459; 56, p. 1008; 58, p. 492)

16 Musculoskeletal System

DIRECTIONS (Questions 751–775): Each of the questions or incomplete statements below is followed by four or five suggested answers or completions. Select the **one** that is best in each case.

751. Gross positional deformity in acute hand injury suggests
    A. nerve bundle compression
    B. tendon or bone injury
    C. soft tissue trauma
    D. vascular compromise
    E. malingering

752. Carpal tunnel syndrome is characterized by
    A. pain in the dorsum of the affected joint
    B. atrophy in the radial nerve distribution
    C. numbness in the median nerve distribution
    D. aggravation of symptoms with wrist in neutral position
    E. most frequent occurrence in young men

753. Shoulder dislocation is **MOST** often
  - **A.** anterior, caused by forced abduction and external rotation
  - **B.** posterior, caused by seizures
  - **C.** posterior, caused by posterior trauma to shoulder
  - **D.** anterior, caused by blunt coronal trauma
  - **E.** inferior, caused by flexion, internal rotation

754. Important features of care for forearm fractures include
  - **A.** awareness of intact vascular and nerve supply
  - **B.** alignment of length and rotation of fragments
  - **C.** assessment of wrist and elbow for injury
  - **D.** limitation of supination and pronation in recovery
  - **E.** all of the above

755. The single **MOST** important bony complication of femoral neck fracture is
  - **A.** fat embolism
  - **B.** restricted range of motion
  - **C.** pain
  - **D.** avascular necrosis
  - **E.** hypercalcinosis

756. A greenstick fracture is seen in children when
  - **A.** calcium intake is inadequate for maturation
  - **B.** one side of bone bows, while the opposing side fractures
  - **C.** primary ossification center arrests growth
  - **D.** tibia resists fracture when fibula fractures
  - **E.** sheering forces tear collateral ligaments of adjacent joint

757. Growth plate fractures
  - **A.** occur in the active chondroblast layer
  - **B.** always result in misdirected growth
  - **C.** may be identified by the Salter Harris classification
  - **D.** cannot have malunion from misdirected growth
  - **E.** do not occur as a crush-type injury

758. The child with congenital hip dislocation
   A. presents with femoral head below the acetabulum
   B. will develop a correct hip if untreated
   C. does not risk permanent deformity
   D. may be classified as teratologic or acquired
   E. is usually male

759. Constitutional chronic illness symptoms associated with inflammatory illness include
   A. fever
   B. nausea
   C. headache
   D. double vision
   E. weight gain

760. Asymmetric bony hypertrophy of the small joints of the fingers is seen in
   A. gout
   B. pseudogout
   C. septic arthritis
   D. osteoarthritis
   E. fibrositis

761. Synovial hypertrophy is **MOST** often associated with
   A. fibrositis
   B. systemic lupus erythematosus
   C. rheumatoid arthritis
   D. pseudogout
   E. dermatomyositis

762. Larger effusions of the knee capsule are **BEST** determined by
   A. ballottement
   B. total aspiration
   C. radiograph
   D. bulge test
   E. Baker's flexion sign

763. Abnormal curvature of the spine
    A. causes in "list" and pelvic tilt
    B. is always correlated with scoliosis
    C. is the presenting sign of ankylosing spondylitis
    D. cannot be caused by muscle spasm
    E. is defined as a deviation angle greater than 15°

764. Skin rash on the face, pericarditis, and glomerulonephritis are signs of
    A. pseudogout
    B. dermatomyositis
    C. dystrophic myopathy
    D. systemic lupus erythematosus
    E. Sjogren's syndrome

765. Patients with acute nongonococcal arthritis
    A. do not usually have underlying illness
    B. usually have *Staphylococcus* in several joints
    C. have infection in previously damaged joints
    D. usually have elevated synovial fluid glucose
    E. may be confirmed by blood culture

766. Lyme disease characteristics include
    A. recurrent inflammatory arthritis
    B. arthritis without fever, rash, or myalgia
    C. absence of neurologic symptoms
    D. spirochetes isolated from synovium
    E. all of the above

767. American Rheumatism Association criteria for rheumatoid arthritis include
    A. morning stiffness
    B. pain on motion or tenderness of at least one joint
    C. soft tissue swelling of at least one joint
    D. synovial histologic changes
    E. all of the above

768. Clinical subsets of rheumatoid arthritis include
   A. Felty's syndrome
   B. Carmichael's syndrome
   C. Sjogren's syndrome
   D. A and C
   E. none of the above

769. Generally recognized side-effects of salicylates used for arthritis treatment include
   A. tinnitus, anemia, gastritis
   B. photophobia, hypercalcemia
   C. pyuria, tinnitus, polyphagia
   D. nasal polyposis, decreased BUN
   E. none of the above

770. Nonsteroidal drugs (NASIDS) used for arthritis treatment cause
   A. analgesic effects
   B. antipyretic effects
   C. antiinflammatory effects
   D. all of the above
   E. none of the above

771. Children who present with classic "Still's disease onset" of rheumatic disease will have
   A. leukopenia, hypothermia, pallor
   B. polyarthritis, high fever, skin rash
   C. high fever, diarrhea, leukopenia
   D. leukocytosis, splenomegaly, hypotheruria
   E. rhinitis leukopenia, uveitis

772. The seronegative spondyloarthropathies share which of the following characteristics?
   A. Presence of inflammatory polyarthritis
   B. Absence of rheumatoid factor
   C. Presence of sacroiliitis
   D. Presence of characteristic nonarticular manifestation
   E. All of the above

773. The **MOST** important pathogenic factor in osteoarthritis is
   A. heredity
   B. age
   C. occupation
   D. trauma
   E. medical history

774. The necrotizing vasculitis clinical syndrome group includes
   A. Wegener's granulomatosis
   B. polymyalgia rheumatica
   C. giant cell arteritis
   D. polyarteritis nodosa
   E. all of the above

775. Signs and symptoms of thoracic outlet syndrome include
   A. increased pain with uplifted arms
   B. paresthesias with elbow flexion
   C. syncope on deep inspiration
   D. sternocleidomastoid spasm
   E. bicipital adhesion

DIRECTIONS (Questions 776–785): The group of questions below consists of lettered headings followed by a list of numbered words, phrases, or statements. For each numbered word, phrase, or statement, select the **one** lettered heading that is most closely associated with it. Each lettered heading may be selected once, more than once, or not at all.

Questions 776–781: Match the accompanying process to each of the following characteristics.
   A. Rheumatoid arthritis
   B. Osteoarthritis
   C. Systemic lupus erythematosus
   D. Ankylosing spondylitis
   E. Gout

776. Bilateral symmetrical polyarthritis

777. Accompanied by inflammatory bowel disease, most frequently in males

778. Joint pain which worsens with activity

779. Results from repetitive occupational activity

780. Mucosal ulcerations of nose and mouth occur

781. Explosive onset

Questions 782–785: Match the following synovial fluid findings to their appropriate etiology.
- **A.** Monosodium urate crystals
- **B.** Calcium pyrophosphate dihydrate crystals
- **C.** *Gonococcus* sp.
- **D.** Malignant cells
- **E.** Eosinophils

782. Cancer

783. Gout

784. Septic arthritis

785. Pseudogout

Explanatory Answers

751. B. The acutely injured hand with positional deformity strongly suggests tendon or bone disruption secondary to the injury. Nerve damage should be assessed by sensory exam. Soft tissue injury will be evidenced by swelling without positional deformity. Vascular compromise will be noted by absence of coloration. (Ref. 65, p. 191)

752. C. The median nerve is compressed as it traverses the carpal area under the transverse carpal ligament on the volar aspect of the wrist. Paresthesia, pain, atrophy, and decreasing strength of the median nerve innervation are seen most commonly in women aged 30 to 60 with this syndrome. (Ref. 65, p. 199)

753. A. Anterior humeral dislocation is most often seen and is the result of forced abduction and external rotation, often accompanied by a blow to the upper outstretched arm. Posterior dislocation, while very rarely seen, can indeed be the result of a seizure. (Ref. 65, p. 224)

754. E. All of the responses are important considerations in the treatment of forearm fractures. (Ref. 65, p. 235)

755. D. Avascular necrosis occurs in 15% to 35% of all cases of femoral neck fracture, and may take up to two years to become evident on x-ray. (Ref. 65, p. 246)

756. B. The radius and ulna most frequently sustain a greenstick fracture, an incomplete transverse fracture with one intact cortex of bone. This deformity can recur after immobilization, and must be reassessed. (Ref. 65, p. 274)

757. C. Salter classifications I to V are the most common method of grading growth plate fractures, which occur in the calcified cartilage layer, sparing the layer of osteoblasts. Malunion can occur from misdirected growth. (Ref. 65, p. 276)

758. D. Congenital hip dislocation, four times more commonly seen in females, is often devastating if left untreated, resulting in permanent disability. Present in 1 of 1500 births, CDH may be comprised of dislocation or subluxation, and may require surgery for correction. (Ref. 65, p. 281)

759. A. Fever, weight loss, fatigue, and stiffness are commonly associated with rheumatoid arthritis, ankylosing spondylitis, and systemic lupus erythematosus. (Ref. 65, p. 1789)

760. D. Bony proximal interphalangeal hypertrophy of osteoarthritis is asymmetrical, often much worse on one side, and may result in positional deformity. (Ref. 65, p. 1791)

761. C. Synovial proliferation is a characteristic pathologic change of rheumatoid arthritis, as well as granuloma and lymphoid follicles in the synovium, and erosion of articular cartilage. (Ref. 65, p. 1741)

762. A. Ballottement of the patella with the knee extended makes significant effusion of the knee capsule obvious. Care must be taken to restrict the volume of the suprapatellar pouch when balloting. (Ref. 65, p. 1743)

763. A. List of the shoulders and torso, and pelvic tilt demonstrated while standing at rest are typical findings of spinal curvature. Paraspinous spasm, often with tenderness, can create significant abnormal curvature. (Ref. 65, p. 1795)

764. D. SLE may present a baffling picture of incremental multisystemic disease with an elusive etiology. Astute recognition of related clinical events and appropriate diagnostic evaluation leads to its diagnosis. (Ref. 65, p. 1791)

765. C. Acute nongonococcal arthritis due to *S. aureus* is not often isolated from a single joint. Many patients have serious underlying illness or are immunosuppressed. Infection frequently localizes to a joint damaged by chronic arthritis. (Ref. 65, p. 1800)

766. A. Recurrent inflammatory arthritis of Lyme disease follows early typical symptoms of rash, fever, malaise, myalgia, and headache. If left untreated, progression of meningitis, cranial nerve palsies, radiculopathies, and cardiac complications are likely. (Ref. 65, p. 1801)

767. E. All are among the eleven diagnostic criteria of ARA, which also includes subcutaneous nodules, symmetric joint swelling, swelling of one other joint, nodule histologic changes, "poor" mucin precipitate, and decalcification on x-ray. (Ref. 65, p. 1802)

768. D. Felty's syndrome of leukopenia, splenomegaly, and rheumatoid arthritis, and Sjogren's syndrome of dry eyes, dry mouth, and rheumatoid arthritis are the most readily recognized of several subsets of RA. (Ref. 65, p. 1802)

769. A. Salicylates cause acute gastritis, gastric ulceration, anemia, and tinnitus in patients taking doses high enough to provide symptomatic improvement. (Ref. 65, p. 1803)

770. D. All three effects are seen in varying degrees of effectiveness for the four basic categories of NASIDS. (Ref. 65, p. 1803)

771. B. Still's disease, or juvenile rheumatoid arthritis, presents with symmetrical arthritis, high fever, skin rash, hepatomegaly, splenomegaly, and leukocytosis. (Ref. 65, p. 1806)

772. E. All of the characteristics listed are found in the set of illnesses that include juvenile rheumatoid arthritis, ankylosing spondylitis, psoriatic arthritis, Reiter's disease, and the arthritis of inflammatory bowel disease. (Ref. 65, p. 1807)

773. B. Age is the single most important determinant of the onset of osteoarthritis. (Ref. 65, p. 1807)

774. E. Each diagnosis involves either small- or medium-sized vessels in acute and/or chronic inflammatory vasculitis. (Ref. 65, p. 1813)

775. A. Movements which narrow the subclavicular space in the area of the scalenus muscle, causing compression of the brachial plexus, and subclavian circulation elicit symptoms. (Ref. 65, p. 1817)

776. A. Rheumatoid arthritis selectively attacks the nonweightbearing small joints of both extremities, with symmetrical findings. (Ref. 65, p. 1790)

777. D. Ankylosing spondylitis, usually seen in males, is often seen in conjunction with one of several different inflammatory diseases of bowel. (Ref. 65, p. 1790)

778. B. As joint wear increases with activity, inflammation is aggravated in degeneration arthritis, resulting in pain. (Ref. 65, p. 1790)

779. B. Osteoarthritis may occur as a result of repetitive movements of joints during work which creates a pattern of deterioration in the joint. (Ref. 65, p. 1790)

780. C. Systemic lupus erythematosus is associated with nasal and oral ulcers, as well as alopecia and photosensitivity. (Ref. 65, p. 1790)

781. E. Gout has an extremely acute onset of excruciating pain, inflammation, local fever, and swelling. (Ref. 65, p. 1790)

782. D. Malignant cells present in synovial analysis suggest primary or metastatic invasion, and should provoke investigation of those causes. (Ref. 65, p. 1793)

783. A. Urate crystals will be found in the synovial fluid of the gouty joint, and can be recognized by their characteristic appearance. (Ref. 65, p. 1793)

784. C. *Gonococcus* sp. is one of many different bacteria that can be responsible for acute or chronic infectious arthritis. Often highly destructive, appropriate antibiotic therapy must be started promptly. (Ref. 65, p. 1793)

785. B. While closely mimicking gout in clinical presentation, pseudogout most often involves the knees, hips, and shoulders. Chondrocalcinosis is present and calcium pyrophosphate dihydrate crystals are seen in synovial aspirate. (Ref. 65, p. 1793)

17 Pulmonary, Hematology, and Otolaryngology

DIRECTIONS (Questions 786–850): Each of the questions or incomplete statements below is followed by four or five suggested answers or completions. Select the one that is best in each case.

786. The **BEST** initial management of vocal nodules is
   A. antibiotics
   B. antacids
   C. voice therapy
   D. direct laryngoscopy and biopsy
   E. laser vaporization

787. A patient presents to the emergency room with epistaxis and a swollen nose, secondary to a fist fight. The **MOST** important step in the initial management of this patient is
   A. palpation of the nose
   B. examination of the nasal septum
   C. plain films of the nose
   D. CT of the head
   E. sinus films

788. A 76-year-old male presents with longstanding difficulty swallowing all foods, with regurgitation after eating, but denies any aspiration. He denies any significant weight loss. He has a 30-pack/year history of smoking. The indirect laryngeal exam is unremarkable. The **MOST** likely diagnosis would be
   A. globus hystericus
   B. esophageal cancer
   C. Zenker's diverticulum
   D. velopharyngeal insufficiency
   E. basal ganglia stroke

789. In a sinus series, the Water's view is best to visualize the
   A. sphenoid sinus
   B. ethmoid sinus
   C. maxillary sinus
   D. frontal sinus
   E. nasopharynx

790. Epistaxis is a sign of all of the following **EXCEPT**
   A. Kartagener's syndrome
   B. hypertension
   C. Osler-Weber-Rendu disease
   D. juvenile nasopharyngeal angiofibroma
   E. chronic nephritis

791. **MOST** taste papillae on the palate are located
   A. near the uvula
   B. near the incisive foramen
   C. near the free edge of the soft palate
   D. near the junction of the hard and soft palates
   E. on the anterior hard palate

792. In allergic rhinitis, the nasal mucosa **MOST** commonly
   A. is pale and pink
   B. is erythematous and glistening
   C. is blue-gray and cobblestoned
   D. is red and friable
   E. has no characteristic features

793. A hematoma of the auricle is **BEST** managed by
  A. observation
  B. antibiotics and pressure dressings
  C. repeated aspiration and pressure dressings
  D. antibiotics alone

794. Typical clinical findings in a patient with malignant otitis externa include all of the following **EXCEPT**
  A. diabetes mellitus
  B. deep ear pain
  C. cranial nerve palsies
  D. identifiable fungal colonies in the ear canal
  E. granulation tissue in the external auditory canal

795. The differential diagnosis of pulsatile tinnitus includes all of the following **EXCEPT**
  A. a venous hum
  B. A-V malformation
  C. cholesteatoma
  D. carotid aneurysm
  E. glomus tumor

796. Which of the following is **MOST** characteristic of vertigo of a central origin?
  A. Absent caloric response
  B. Abnormal acoustic reflex
  C. Vertical nystagmus
  D. Emesis
  E. Positional nystagmus

797. A 52-year-old white male presents with a painful ulcer of the left lateral tongue. He smokes $2^1/_2$ packs/day and is a social drinker. On physical examination, the patient has a small 1-cm ulcer in the lateral aspect of his left tongue, opposite to a partial dental plate, which is irritating the tongue. The **MOST** appropriate recommendation for this patient would be

A. referral to dermatologist for evaluation and biopsy
B. remove the dentures; start on saline gargles until ulcer heals
C. start a ten-day course of penicillin and then reevaluate the patient
D. stop smoking
E. refer to a dentist and have the plate filed and refitted

798. Facial paralysis in Ramsey-Hunt syndrome is due to which of the following viruses?

A. Herpes simplex
B. Coxsackie
C. Rubella
D. Herpes zoster
E. Epstein-Barr

799. The **BEST** treatment of a nondisplaced, anterior wall frontal sinus fracture is

A. frontal sinus obliteration
B. observation
C. exploration and wire fixation
D. decompression of the frontal sinus
E. Lynch procedure

800. Signs of temporal bone fracture include all of the following **EXCEPT**

A. cerebrospinal otorhinorrhea
B. conductive hearing loss
C. sensorineural hearing loss
D. numbness of the face
E. facial nerve paralysis

801. A shallow type A tympanogram suggests
   A. serous otitis media
   B. eustachian tube dysfunction
   C. ossicular chain fixation
   D. tympanic membrane perforation
   E. tympanosclerosis

802. The **MOST** common organism in acute bacterial sialoadenitis is
   A. *H. influenzae*
   B. beta-hemolytic streptococci
   C. *S. aureus*
   D. *P. aeruginosa*
   E. *S. pneumoniae*

803. A 19-year-old white male, college football player, presents with extremely large hands and feet, and a bilateral temporal visual field defect. He also has von Willebrand's disease. The **BEST** treatment for this patient's problem would be
   A. cerebral angiography and embolization
   B. radiation therapy
   C. transphenoidal hypophysectomy
   D. corrective lenses
   E. factor-8 replacement

804. A common cause of sudden hearing loss is
   A. aural atresia
   B. vestibular neuronitis
   C. cerumen impaction
   D. glomus tumor
   E. cerebrovascular accident

805. Posterior cervical lymphadenopathy is **MOST** often associated with cancer of the
   A. anterior two-thirds of the tongue
   B. posterior one-third of the tongue
   C. true vocal cord
   D. pyriform sinus
   E. nasopharynx

806. In temporal bone fractures, the facial nerve is **MOST** frequently injured in the region of the
   A. porus acusticus
   B. geniculate ganglion
   C. oval window
   D. mastoid segment
   E. stylomastoid foramen

807. Which of the following is **NOT** a symptom of unilateral laryngeal paralysis in adults?
   A. Hoarseness
   B. Aspiration
   C. Ineffective cough
   D. Stridor
   E. Impaired valsalva

808. Which of the following is an occupational hazard of nickel and wood workers?
   A. Inverting papilloma
   B. Squamous cell carcinoma of the nasal vestibule
   C. Nasal polyposis
   D. Nasal adenocarcinoma
   E. Silicosis

809. Which of the following has **NOT** been implicated in the production of otitis media with effusion?
   A. Adenoid hypertrophy
   B. Sinusitis
   C. Upper respiratory tract infection
   D. Allergy
   E. External otitis

810. While scuba diving, a patient noticed a sudden pop in his right ear, and now he is dizzy and cannot hear well on the right. The **MOST** likely diagnosis is
   A. stapes fracture
   B. semicircular canal fracture
   C. tympanic membrane rupture
   D. round window rupture
   E. otitis externa

811. A 56-year-old singer presents with four weeks of hoarseness. He has smoked one pack of cigarettes per day for forty years. Physical examination shows a nodular mass on his left vocal fold. Management should consist of

   A. voice rest for two weeks
   B. voice therapy for six months
   C. antacids
   D. antibiotics
   E. direct laryngoscopy and biopsy

812. A 30-year-old woman complains of severe nasal obstruction, relieved only by topical Neo-Synephrine. The **MOST** important step in managing this patient is

   A. sinus films
   B. allergy testing
   C. administration of steroids
   D. discontinuation of nasal spray
   E. chest x-ray

813. Which of the following audiometric findings is characteristic of otosclerosis with fixation of the stapes?

   A. Type B tympanogram
   B. Type IV Betsy tracing
   C. Rollover of PB function
   D. Absent acoustic reflex
   E. PTA of 5 dB

814. A 30-year-old male develops a sore throat, which gradually increases in severity over a few days. He presents to the emergency room with a sore throat, dysphagia, trismus, and mild airway obstruction. His **MOST** likely diagnosis is

   A. carcinoma of the pharynx
   B. parotitis
   C. peritonsillar abscess
   D. epiglottitis
   E. Vincent's angina

815. A sequela of faulty facial nerve regeneration is
   A. anosmia
   B. synkinesis
   C. inadequate saliva
   D. facial numbness
   E. dysphagia

816. Pneumatic otoscopy is useful for detecting
   A. tympanosclerosis
   B. otosclerosis
   C. bullous myringitis
   D. sensorineural hearing loss
   E. otitis media

817. The **MOST** common cause of bilateral vocal fold paralysis is
   A. carcinoma of the lung
   B. thyroidectomy
   C. radical neck dissection
   D. laryngeal papillomatosis
   E. amyotrophic lateral sclerosis

818. A two-year-old child is brought to the emergency room by his parents after he was found with an open bottle of caustic substance. He has erythema of the oral mucosa and is drooling. The appropriate emergency management should be
   A. Ipecac to induce vomiting
   B. gastric lavage
   C. observation only
   D. immediate endoscopy
   E. barium swallow

819. Medical management of Meniere's disease includes
   A. anticonvulsants
   B. diuretics
   C. antihypertensives
   D. antibiotics
   E. neuroleptics

820. A 50-year-old male has shown no signs of recurrence for two years following radiation therapy of a T1, squamous carcinoma. He is at **GREATEST** risk for
   A. cervical metastasis
   B. distant metastasis
   C. recurrence of the tumor
   D. a second primary tumor
   E. radionecrosis of the larynx

821. A 24-year-old male was involved as a passenger in an automobile accident, striking his head on the windshield. In the emergency room, he is hoarse and mildly stridorous, and palpation of the cervical skin yields a "crackling" sensation. His vital signs are stable and he is in no acute distress. The **NEXT** step in his management should be
   A. computerized tomography of the neck
   B. barium swallow
   C. close observation
   D. tracheotomy
   E. intubation

822. Approximately 15% of patients afflicted with Bell's palsy will undergo complete degeneration. Return of some facial movement should be expected within
   A. one month
   B. three months
   C. six months
   D. one year
   E. two years

823. The **MOST** common malignant tumor of the parotid gland is
   A. Warthin's tumor
   B. adenoid cystic
   C. pleomorphic adenoma
   D. mucoepidermoid
   E. oncocytoma

824. Hyperosmia may result from
   A. Kallmann's syndrome
   B. an upper respiratory infection
   C. untreated Addison's disease
   D. nasal septal deviation
   E. chronic sinusitis

825. Abnormalities of the pinna are commonly associated with hearing impairment. The impairment is usually secondary to
   A. sensorineural damage
   B. otosclerosis
   C. recurrent ear infections
   D. absence of the ossicles
   E. malformed ossicles

826. Nasal polyps in children are frequently seen in association with
   A. Still's disease
   B. juvenile onset diabetes mellitus
   C. cystic fibrosis
   D. acute glomerulonephritis

827. A person with epistaxis has posterior and anterior packs in place. He continues to bleed copiously, despite this treatment. The **NEXT** step would be
   A. hypotensive therapy
   B. placement of larger packs
   C. cauterization of Little's area
   D. surgical intervention
   E. embolization of the bleeding vessel

828. You are asked to evaluate an infant with noisy respirations. The infant has a moderate amount of stridor, which is biphasic and more pronounced when the infant cries. The child nurses without difficulty. The child **MOST** likely has
   A. choanal atresia
   B. epiglottis
   C. laryngomalacia
   D. laryngeal web
   E. subglottic hemangioma

829. The **MOST** common presentation of an acoustic neuroma is
   A. sudden hearing loss
   B. gradual hearing loss
   C. sudden onset of vertigo
   D. gradual onset of vertigo
   E. fluctuating vertigo

830. Patients who receive cochlear implants experience which of the following hearing results?
   A. Normal hearing
   B. Improved pure tone average
   C. Conductive hearing loss
   D. Tinnitus
   E. Awareness of environmental sounds

831. Which of the following is **NOT** useful in evaluating hearing in infants?
   A. Auditory brainstem responses
   B. Crib-o-gram audiometry
   C. Pure tone audiometry
   D. Acoustic reflex
   E. Tympanometry

832. A 70-year-old black male admitted for evaluation of low-back pain is found to have bone x-rays with multiple lytic lesions of the skull and pelvis, with a total serum protein of 12 g/dL. The **MOST** likely diagnosis is
   A. acute lymphoblastic leukemia
   B. multiple myeloma
   C. Hodgkin's disease
   D. chronic myelogenous leukemia
   E. chronic lymphocytic leukemia

833. A 25-year-old white male presents with a three-month history of painless enlargement of bilateral cervical lymph nodes, fever, and night sweats. The **MOST** probable diagnosis is
   A. acute lymphoblastic leukemia
   B. multiple myeloma
   C. Hodgkin's disease
   D. chronic myelogenous leukemia
   E. chronic lymphocytic leukemia

834. A 56-year-old black female admitted for evaluation of fatigue and abdominal discomfort is found to have a mass in the left upper quadrant, consistent with an enlarged spleen; a hematocrit of 27%; white blood cell count of 150,000, with 55% segmented neutrophils; 15% band forms; 10% metamyelocytes; 10% myelocytes; 2% promyelocytes; 3% eosinophils and 5% basophils; and a platelet count of 850,000. The **MOST** likely diagnosis is

A. acute lymphoblastic leukemia
B. multiple myeloma
C. Hodgkin's disease
D. chronic myelogenous leukemia
E. chronic lymphocytic leukemia

835. A 65-year-old white male was evaluated preoperatively for inguinal hernia repair. A routine CBC showed a hematocrit of 45%, hemoglobin 14.0 g/dL, white blood cell count of 70,000, and platelet of count of 250,000. The differential revealed 10% segmented neutrophils and 90% mature small lymphocytes. The **MOST** likely diagnosis is

A. acute lymphoblastic leukemia
B. multiple myeloma
C. Hodgkin's disease
D. chronic myelogenous leukemia
E. chronic lymphocytic leukemia

836. A recently jaundiced, 25-year-old black man was found to have a hematocrit of 32%. Laboratory studies revealed a low reticulocyte count (0.5%) and elevated levels of SGOT, SGPT, and LDH. When you see him two weeks later, all lab tests are unchanged. The **LEAST** likely cause of his anemia is

A. G-6-PD deficiency
B. sickle cell anemia
C. autoimmune hemolytic anemia
D. paroxysmal nocturnal hemoglobinuria

837. A 25-year-old white male college student noticed the appearance of enlarged nontender bilateral cervical lymphadenopathy. He had not had fever, weight loss, night sweats, nor a sore throat. The hematocrit, platelet, white blood cell, and differential counts were normal. Which one of the following is the **MOST** likely diagnosis?
    A. Infectious mononucleosis
    B. Chronic lymphocytic leukemia
    C. Hodgkin's disease
    D. Multiple myeloma

838. Which of the following tests would be **MOST** likely to give a definitive diagnosis in the above case?
    A. Mono spot test
    B. Lymph node biopsy
    C. Bone marrow examination
    D. Serum protein electrophoresis

839. Which one of the following is **FALSE** concerning iron deficiency anemia?
    A. Men presenting with iron deficiency should have a careful evaluation of blood loss
    B. Reticulocytosis is not present in untreated iron deficiency
    C. Serum ferritin, when 12 mg/mL is indicative of iron deficiency
    D. Hypochromic, microcytic red blood cells are a specific finding

840. A 60-year-old black man has constipation. Routine laboratory studies reveal mild anemia (hematocrit 36%). The serum iron is low, serum ferritin is low, total iron binding capacity is high, and initial stool guaiac is negative. The **MOST** important next step is
    A. improve the patient's nutritional habits
    B. begin iron therapy
    C. GI tract evaluation (x-rays and endoscopy)
    D. hemoglobin electrophoresis
    E. tests for iron malabsorption

841. A 27-year-old black female experienced the onset of weakness and easy bruisability. CBC shows HCT 23%, WBC 30,000 with 75% "immature cells," and platelet count 15,000. Which of the following is **NOT** a likely diagnosis?
    A. Acute myeloblastic leukemia
    B. Acute lymphoblastic leukemia
    C. Chronic lymphocytic leukemia
    D. Acute monoblastic leukemia

842. A young woman has mild anemia. The peripheral blood smear shows generalized microcytosis and hypochromia. Serum iron is 70 (normal 60 to 130), iron binding capacity 325 (normal 275 to 350) and ferritin 40 (normal 30 to 200). The reticulocyte count is low. The **NEXT** step should be
    A. therapy with iron
    B. GI evaluation
    C. bone marrow exam
    D. hemoglobin A2 quantitation
    E. serum B_{12} and folate levels

843. All of the following are true about iron deficiency **EXCEPT**
    A. spoon nails and angular stomatitis are physical findings in some patients
    B. serum total iron-binding capacity is elevated
    C. treatment with $FeSO_4$ results in reticulocytosis in 5 to 10 days
    D. patients seldom complain of peculiar dietary cravings

844. A young woman is found to have a mild anemia with normocytic, normochromic indices and reticulopenia. Which of the following would **MOST** likely reveal the cause of anemia?
    A. Serum iron and iron binding capacity
    B. Serum B_{12} and folate levels
    C. GI evaluation
    D. Hemoglobin A2 quantitation

845. The **MOST** important indication of hemolysis is
    A. abnormal red cell morphology
    B. reticulocytosis without blood loss
    C. direct bilirubinemia
    D. hematuria

846. The normal response to hemolysis does **NOT** include
A. early release of reticulocytes from the marrow
B. polychromatophilic red blood cells on peripheral blood
C. splenic sequestration of abnormal red blood cells
D. reduced folate requirements

847. An elderly woman presents with complaints of shortness of breath and general malaise. Her hematocrit is 20 and her reticulocyte count is 4.0% (uncorrected). Her peripheral blood smear shows macrocytosis and hypersegmented polys. A quick check of her MCV reveals that it is 120 U^3. Which of the following tests is **LEAST** appropriate in this situation?
A. Serum B_{12} folate levels
B. Schilling's test
C. Thorough neurological examination
D. Therapeutic trial of folate alone

848. Causes of increased platelet destruction, producing thrombocytopenia, include all of the following **EXCEPT**
A. immune thrombocytopenic purpura
B. folic acid deficiency
C. liver disease with splenomegaly
D. disseminated intravascular coagulation
E. aortic valve prosthesis

849. A patient with osteomyelitis has been treated for a prolonged time with antibiotics. The patient has no bleeding history, but has been a heavy alcohol user for years. The PT and PTT are found to be prolonged; while adding aged serum to the patient plasma seems to correct these abnormalities. The diagnostic possibilities include
A. folate deficiency
B. vitamin K deficiency
C. fibrinogen deficiency
D. hypocalcemia
E. hypersplenism

850. The **MOST** likely diagnosis in a ten-year-old Oriental boy with a hematocrit of 20%, reticulocyte count of 20%, MCV 69, peripheral smear showing numerous target cells with poikilocytosis, skull x-rays showing a "crew-cut" appearance, and splenomegaly on physical exam is
    A. anemia of chronic disease
    B. sickle cell disease
    C. thalassemia major
    D. paroxysmal nocturnal hemoglobinuria

Explanatory Answers

786. C. Vocal nodules are usually bilateral, and situated at the junction of the anterior and middle thirds of the vocal cords, and frequently seen in patients who use their voices professionally, eg, singers. The best initial management is voice therapy to deal with the vocal dysfunction that may be present. (Ref. 66, p. 621)

787. B. Epistaxis secondary to nasal trauma typically involves the anterior septum in younger individuals, and more posterior sites with increasing age. The initial step in the management of epistaxis involves identifying the site of bleeding. (Ref. 67, p. 314)

788. C. Dysphasia with regurgitation of food that is undigested after a meal suggests a pulsion or Zenker's diverticulum, though it must be distinguished from other pharyngeal diverticula. (Ref. 68, pp. 582–585)

789. C. Conventional plain film remains the best screening study for assessing paranasal sinuses and facial bones, with the posteroanterior occipitomental projection (Water's view) best demonstrating the maxillary sinuses. (Ref. 67, p. 225)

790. A. Kartagener's syndrome is a disorder of primary ciliary dysfunction, often referred to as immobile cilia syndrome, that alters mucociliary clearance. The diagnosis is made by light or electron microscopic examination of a nasal smear taken from the medial surface of a turbinate. (Ref. 69, pp. 985–991)

791. D. The taste papillae on the palate for sour (acid and bitter) taste are located near the junction of the hard and soft palates. (Ref. 67, p. 363)

792. C. The nasal, oral, and facial signs of allergic rhinitis include the characteristic "allergic salute" shiners under the eyes, gaping open-mouthed appearance, and grayish, mucous covered nasal mucosa. (Ref. 70)

793. C. Auricular hematoma secondary to direct trauma usually occurs beneath the perichondrium and produces excruciating pain, as a space-occupying lesion. Failure to aspirate and control bleeding can lead to suppuration of the hematoma and cartilage necrosis, or thickening and scarring of the cartilage, commonly known as "cauliflower ear." (Ref. 71, pp. 881–885)

794. D. Malignant necrotizing external otitis is a serious infection caused by *P. aeruginosa* in elderly diabetics, manifest by active granulation tissue in the external auditory canal, pain on movement of the temporomandibular joint, and marked tenderness on palpation beneath the external ear canal. (Ref. 72, pp. 1257–1294)

795. C. Pulsatile tinnitus is a sign characteristic of vascular (glomus) tumors, whereas cholesteatoma, comprised of keratinizing stratified squamous epithelium, present with cranial nerve symptomatology, sensorineural hearing loss, or laryngopharyngeal dysfunction. (Ref. 67, p. 173)

796. C. Disorders of the vestibular system result in the illusion of movement (vertigo), as well as imbalance and disordered eye movements (nystagmus). Central lesions produce vertical (direction-changing) nystagmus on position testing. (Ref. 66, p. 432)

797. A. Most lingual cancers involve the lateral surface of the oral tongue with individuals typically complaining of infrequent pain or a mass noted while chewing. Squamous cell carcinoma involving the oral cavity is six times greater in smokers, and 15 times greater if the individual also drinks. Because of the risk factors present, the course of action should be that of biopsy. (Ref. 67, p. 386)

798. D. Ramsey-Hunt syndrome manifest by facial paralysis, swelling and vesiculation of the external auditory canal, intense pain, vertigo, and sensorineural deafness is due to herpes zoster. (Ref. 73, pp. 1853–1878)

799. B. Anterior wall frontal sinus fractures are often secondary to vehicular or industrial accidents, or blunt trauma from assault with a weapon. According to the management protocol for frontal sinus fractures proposed by Shockley et al, the treatment of choice is observation. (Ref. 74, pp. 18–22)

800. D. Fracture of the temporal bone, whether longitudinal, transverse, or mixed, can produce injury to the tympanic membrane, ossicular disruption, hematoma, disruption of the labyrinthine capsule, and dural tears, resulting in cerebrospinal fluid otorrhea, facial nerve paralysis, hearing impairment, and pain. Sensation of the face is, however, provided by the trigeminal nerve, which follows a course separate from the facial nerve (CN7). (Ref. 67, p. 93)

801. C. Tympanometry assesses the mobility of the membrane and middle ear (ossicular) system. The shallow type A tympanogram suggests ossicular fixation, in contrast to membrane damage. (Ref. 67, pp. 44–46)

802. C. Acute bacterial sialadenitis secondary to *S. aureus* results from stasis of the saliva due to decreased production and increased viscosity, allowing for the growth of pathogens. It is characterized by erythema, pain, tenderness, swelling, and a purulent discharge from Stensen's duct. (Ref. 67, p. 377)

803. C. Effective surgical treatment of a pituitary adenoma with encroachment on the optic nerves involves a transphenoidal approach to the pituitary gland with a sublabial incision leading to hypophysectomy. (Ref. 67, p. 727)

804. C. The sudden appearance of a conductive hearing loss is typically due to an obstructing ear canal lesion. Cerumen impaction of the external canal is the most frequent cause of such loss. (Ref. 66, p. 154)

805. E. Lymphatic flow and presumably metastatic cell migration is generally downward medially and posteriorly toward the mediastinum, with the upper nodes most commonly involved in metastasis. The posterior cervical drains the nasopharynx, oropharynx, supraglottic larynx, and hypopharynx. (Ref. 67, p. 487)

806. B. Temporal bone fracture of the transverse or mixed type that transect the petrous pyramid disrupt the integrity of the facial nerve in the area of the geniculate ganglion within the internal auditory meatus. (Ref. 67, p. 18)

807. D. Unilateral laryngeal paralysis presents acutely with hoarseness. Less commonly reported symptoms include ineffective cough, aspiration secondary to loss of laryngeal sensation, and impaired valsalva due to inability to approximate cords for closure. Stridor, by contrast, is a manifestation of airway obstruction or impedance to air flow. (Ref. 67, p. 658)

808. D. Etiologic factors for primary adenocarcinoma and the nasal cavities include chronic sinusitis, nasal polyposis, and smoking, with an increased incidence of appearance in woodworkers and persons exposed to nickel and cadmium. (Ref. 75, p. 625)

809. E. Infections of the external auditory canal without the presence of a perforated tympanic membrane to facilitate extension to the middle ear are not associated with otitis media with effusion. (Ref. 66, p. 636)

810. D. Compressive inward pressure on the tympanic membrane gets transferred to the stapes attached to the oval window, with further amplification resulting in round window rupture, endolymph movement causing dizziness, and disruption of the organ of corti, producing hearing loss. (Ref. 67, p. 63)

811. E. A nodular mass on a vocal fold in a symptomatic individual with a 40-pack/year history of smoking should be managed first by direct visualization and biopsy of the mass lesion, as malignancy is to be suspected until proven otherwise. (Ref. 67, p. 647)

812. D. Commonly used vasoconstrictors such as 3% ephedrine sulfate solution, 1% phenylephrine hydrochloride (Neo-Synephrine), and oxymetazoline (Afrin) must be used with caution, as their use is associated with tachycardia, rebound congestion, and chemical instability. Repeated use can lead, within days, to paradoxical vasodilation and soft tissue swelling, best managed by discontinuation of the nasal spray. (Ref. 76)

813. D. Stapedial fixation with progressive hearing loss is the result of abnormal bone replacement due to the genetic disorder otosclerosis. Absence of the acoustic (stapedial) reflex is indicative of a conductive hearing loss. The acoustic reflex is measured using a probe sealed in the ear canal, where ipsilateral reviewed sound produces contraction of the stapedial muscles and a change in the stiffness of the middle ear system. (Ref. 67, p. 46)

814. C. Both squamous cell carcinoma and suppurative tonsillitis may perforate the tonsillar capsule. In tonsillitis, the persistence of and lateralization of the sore throat to one side, with increasing pharyngeal pain, dysphasia, trismus, copious secretions, plus swelling of the tonsil and soft palate suggests peritonsillar abscess. (Ref. 67, p. 410)

815. B. The facial nerve is responsible for activation of the muscles of facial expression, with faulty nerve regeneration following trauma or surgery producing synkinesis. (Ref. 67, pp. 831–832)

816. E. Pneumatic otoscopy yields information about the mobility of the tympanic membrane, with the presence of pus, blood, or serum in the middle ear retarding membrane movement. (Ref. 67, p. 30)

817. B. The inferior thyroid artery, as it crosses medically, posterior to the common carotid artery, comes in close proximity to the recurrent laryngeal nerve. Knowledge of this relationship is essential during thyroidectomy to avoid nerve severance, leading to bilateral vocal fold paralysis. (Ref. 67, p. 461)

818. D. Ingestion of caustic substances produces extensive mucosal damage, specifically burns and drooling. Immediate endoscopy is indicated to determine the presence of burns, but should not extend through a burned area, to avoid perforation. (Ref. 67, p. 536)

819. B. The predominant histologic lesion of Meniere's disease is an increase in the volume of endolymph, causing a bowing displacement of Reissner's membrane into the scala vestibuli. The initial management is medical, usually involving some form of salt restriction, diuretic, and vestibular suppressant. Diuretic therapy is used with intent to reduce body fluid retention on the premise that it correlates with hydropic changes in the labyrinth. (Ref. 67, p. 104)

820. D. A T1 lesion is less than or equal to two centimeters with no node involvement or other metastasis. Individuals treated with radiation therapy are at risk of developing a second primary tumor. (Ref. 67, pp. 385–386)

821. D. Blunt or penetrating trauma may cause acute airway obstruction and respiratory distress. Inspiratory stridor with hoarseness and the presence of subcutaneous emphysema suggest the presence of laryngeal fracture with involvement of the recurrent laryngeal nerve. Endoscopic examination with tracheostomy is indicated. (Ref. 67, p. 668)

822. D. Bell's palsy is a sudden, unilateral facial paralysis, without identifiable cause, thought due to a neurotropic infection, with inflammation in the temporal bone facial canal leading to blood supply compression, myelin tube degeneration, and a conduction block neuroplegia.

Approximately 85% will completely recover over a 3- to 4-week period. Another 15% will partially recovery. Where nerve degeneration is involved, some facial movement can be expected by one year's time. (Ref. 77, p. 692)

823. D. Benign tumors of the salivary gland include the pleomorphic adenoma, monomorphic adenoma, Warthin's tumor, and the oncocytoma. Mucoepidermoid carcinoma is malignant, and accounts for 35% of all malignant salivary gland neoplasms and 50% of all parotid malignant tumors. (Ref. 78, p. 396)

824. C. While upper respiratory infections, deviated nasal septum, and chronic sinusitis may temporarily contribute to nasal obstruction and a decreased sense of smell, they do not heighten one's sense of olfaction. It has been observed that individuals with adrenal insufficiency have an increased sense of smell unexplained by the underlying pathophysiology. (Ref. 79, pp. 9–11)

825. E. The auricle of the external ear develops from six mesenchymal swellings, called auricular hillocks, that develop around the dorsal ends of the first and second bronchial grooves. These hillocks fuse to form the auricle. Abnormalities of the pinna, because of its embryological relationship to the first and second bronchial arches, which provide the malleus/incus and stapes, respectively, suggest the possibility of ossicular abnormalities. (Ref. 80, p. 76)

826. C. A review of patients with cystic fibrosis revealed that 10% developed polyps, while 50% of children with polyps had cystic fibrosis. (Ref. 81, pp. 1488–1495)

827. D. Copious nasal epistaxis despite the use of posterior and anterior packing requires considering other than usual causes for bleeding, such as tumors, vascular anomalies, and posttraumatic injuries, plus the use of surgical intervention. (Ref. 67, p. 316)

828. E. Infants with congenital subglottic hemangioma, a rare slow-growing mass, typically develop a diminished cry, biphasic stridor, and poor feeding habits, with symptoms aggravated by crying or respiratory infections. Epiglottis, by contrast, is associated with inspiratory stridor. (Ref. 67, p. 615)

829. B.   Acoustic neuroma is a benign encapsulated tumor that arises most frequently from the vestibular division of the eighth cranial nerve. Compression of the vestibular/or cochlear division results in the characteristic unilateral, progressive sensorineural hearing loss. (Ref. 67, p. 112)

830. E.   Cochlear implants, specifically multichannel systems, are gaining wide acceptance as a major rehabilitative tool for postlingually deafened adults because of the documentation of auditory speech recognition and an awareness of environmental sound. (Ref. 67, pp. 176–182)

831. C.   The most basic hearing test remains pure tone audiometry with signals presented by air conduction (through an earphone) and by bone conduction (through a vibrator applied to the head). A second component of the basic audiometric test comprises the speech reception threshold. Both these techniques are inappropriate for testing infants, as they require an understanding of language, and the ability to process and follow auditory messages and actively participate in the testing process. (Ref. 67, pp. 41–42)

832. B.   Multiple myeloma (plasma cell myeloma) has a peak incidence during the seventh decade of life, and is manifest by bone pain, typically in the back or chest in more than two thirds of individuals, weakness and fatigue, pallor, anemia, hepatomegaly, 20% of patients, and hypercalcemia. (Ref. 82, p. 1027)

833. C.   Hodgkin's disease usually presents with supradiaphragmatic lymph node involvement, and occasionally with generalized lymphatic disease; the median age of diagnosis is 26 to 31 years; it affects the white population; and is predominantly accompanied by an unexplained history of fever and night sweats. (Ref. 82, pp. 921–922)

834. D.   Chronic myeloid leukemia commonly presents as anemia, bleeding, and splenomegaly. Laboratory parameters typically reveal a leukocyte count between 100 and 300×10^9/L, thrombocytosis, and a wide spectrum of immature and mature myeloid cells. (Ref. 82, p. 859)

835. E.   The two time-honored essential requirements to diagnosis of chronic lymphocytic leukemia are (1) a sustained absolute lymphocytosis in peripheral blood, and (2) a lymphocytosis in the bone marrow. The blood lymphocyte count threshold has been set at 10×10^9. No constitutional symptoms are exhibited, with laboratory studies revealing an absolute lymphocytosis with a differential cell count of lymphocytes ranging from 30% to 99% of all nucleated cells. (Ref. 82, pp. 991–992)

836. C. Persons with increased red blood cell tumors due to acute blood loss, sequestration, or hemolysis usually have anemia and an elevated reticulocyte count. The low reticulocyte count in the presence of elevated enzymes suggests hepatocellular disease as the cause of the nonmegaloblastic anemia. (Ref. 82, p. 308)

837. C. Hodgkin's disease is a problem most often of young adult white males that presents as bilateral lymph node enlargement, supradiaphragmatic in origin. (Ref. 82, pp. 921–923)

838. B. The initial step of staging Hodgkin's disease is the lymph node biopsy, along with biopsy confirmation of other abnormal sites, such as liver or bone. (Ref. 82, p. 922)

839. D. As hemoglobin production becomes restored, iron deficiency anemia develops, resulting in a gradual replacement of normocytic, lyponormocytic red cells by normochronic red cells with a microcytic, hypochromic population. Both the time needed to replace the female population and the extent of disparity believing erythroid needs and available iron supply determine the rate of change. (Ref. 85, p. 337)

840. C. The presence of iron loss depletion due to either metabolism or blood loss in an elderly person with a gastrointestinal problem initially warrants GI tract evaluation as the next step in determining the cause of the abnormal laboratory parameters. (Ref. 82, p. 337)

841. C. The anemia, bruisability, and thrombocytopemia with immature cells on differential count mitigates against chronic lymphocytic leukemia, which requires an absolute lymphocytosis with a threshold count of 10×10^9, along with a differential cell count of lymphocytes (not immature cells) ranging from 30% to 99%. (Ref. 82, p. 99)

842. D. The peripheral blood smear showing generalized microcytosis and hypochromia is highly suggestive of iron deficiency, but is not borne out by the laboratory evaluation of iron status. The observation of importance is the anemia and low reticulocyte count, suggesting inadequate red blood cell production, in this case inadequate hemoglobin synthesis. The next step to ascertain the cause of the microcytic anemia is hemoglobin electrophoresis to assist in defining a potential thalassemia trait, followed by bone marrow examination. (Ref. 82, p. 307)

843. D. In all ages and sexes, but particularly in pregnant women and children, pica, the compulsive chewing or ingestion of food or nonfood substances, may contribute to iron deficiency if the material ingested inhibits iron absorption. (Ref. 82, p. 336)

844. D. Anemia with reticulopenia irrespective of cell indices, in this case, normocytosis and normochromia, suggests inadequate/inappropriate hemoglobin synthesis, which requires hemoglobin electrophoresis. (Ref. 82, p. 337)

845. B. The feedback control system of erythropoiesis provides the basis for the replenishment of approximately 0.8% of the red blood cell pool on a daily basis, with young erythrocytes released from the marrow. These reticulocytes are larger than mature RBCs, plus their number permits an assessment of the marrow's response to peripheral anemia. When the cause of anemia is blood loss or hemolytic destruction in the periphery, erythropoietin overload of the marrow leads to reticulocytosis. (Ref. 82, p. 303)

846. D. Since folate is necessary for hematopoiesis, folate requirements are increased when there is (1) significant compensating erythopoiesis in response to red blood cell destruction, (2) abnormal hematopoiesis, or (3) inhibition by abnormal cells in the marrow. (Ref. 82, p. 410)

847. D. The presentation is one of megaloblastic anemia with a compensation reticulocytosis in response to abnormal hematopoiesis, and cardiopulmonary syndrome, resulting in an approximate 50% reduction in the hemoglobin condition. The exact cause of the megaloblastic anemia must be determined before initiating any therapy. (Ref. 82, pp. 412–413)

848. B. Thrombocytopenia caused by increased platelet destruction develops when the rate of platelet destruction overcomes the ability of the bone marrow to produce platelets. The causes of such destruction are both immune- and nonimmune-related. The nonimmunologic causes to consider include bypass surgery, renal transplant, bone marrow transplantation, hemolytic anemia syndrome, thrombotic thrombocytopenia purpura, and disseminated intravascular coagulation. (Ref. 82, p. 1502)

849. B.   Vitamin K plays a critical role in the posttranslation modifications of the blood coagulation proteins, factor VII, factor IX, factor X, prothrombin, and the plasma anticoagulants. Proteins C and S are absorbed in the ilium; thus fat-soluble vitamins can be interfered with at the absorptive stage, in the presence of enterohepatic circulation defects due to biliary disease. The history of chronic alcohol ingestion and that of antibiotics suggest either a malabsorption syndrome or vitamin K antagonism, as antibiotics such as maxalactim and cefamandole can cause hypoprothrombinemia. (Ref. 82, p. 1374)

850. C.   Thalassemias are inherited and encountered in virtually any ethnic group, being more common in the Mediterranean basin and equational regions of Asia and Africa. The discolor and impaired globin biosynthesis is characterized by severe microcytosis; bizarre poikilocytes, target cells, and nucleated red blood cells; a low retriculocyte count; and hypercellularity of the bone marrow. The sinking changes in the skull and facial bones include thickening of the frontal bone, with perpendicular bony trabeculae appearing as "hair-on-end," due to the hypertrophy and expansion of the marrow with widening of the marrow space. (Ref. 82, pp. 375–376)

References

1. Tanagho EA, McAninch JW, eds: *Smith's General Urology,* ed 12. Norwalk, CT, Appleton and Lange, 1988.

2. Craig CR, Stitzel RE: *Modern Pharmacology,* ed 3. Boston, Little, Brown and Co, 1990.

3. Sanford JP: *Guide to Antimicrobial Therapy 1990.* West Bethesda, MD, Antimicrobial Therapy, Inc, 1990.

4. Waldinger RJ: *Psychiatry for Medical Students.* Washington, DC, American Psychiatric Association, 1984.

5. Kane RL, Ouslander JG, Abrass IB: *Essentials of Clinical Geriatrics,* ed 2. New York, McGraw-Hill, 1989.

6. *Guide to Clinical Preventive Services: Report of the U.S. Preventive Services Task Force.* Baltimore, Williams and Wilkins, 1989.

7. *Scientific American Medicine, Vol 2,* Chapter 13, Section VI, 1990.

8. Wilson JD et al (eds): *Harrison's Principles of Internal Medicine,* ed 12. New York, McGraw-Hill, 1991.

9. Katzung BG (ed): *Basic and Clinical Pharmacology,* ed 4. Norwalk, CT, Appleton and Lange, 1989.

10. *Morbidity and Mortality Weekly Report*, Vol 38, No 10, March 17, 1989.

11. Chasnoff IJ, Burns, KA, Burns WJ: Cocaine use in pregnancy: Perinatal morbidity and mortality. *Neurotoxicology and Teratology* 1987;9:291–293.

12. Mandell GL, Douglas RG, Bennett JE: *Principles and Practice of Infectious Diseases.* New York, Churchill Livingstone, 1990.

13. Muma RD, Borucki MJ, Lyons BA, Pollard RB: Evaluation of patients infected with human immunodeficiency virus type 1, part I: History and physical examination. *Physician Assistant* 1991;15[1]:23–32.

14. Muma RD, Borucki MJ, Lyons BA, Pollard RB: Evaluation of patients infected with human immunodeficiency virus type 1, part II: Diagnostic and psychosocial evaluation. *Physician Assistant* 1991;15[2]:15,19–22.

15. Fischl MA, Richman DD, Hansen N et al: The safety and efficacy of Zidovudine (AZT) in the treatment of subjects with mildly symptomatic human immunodeficiency virus type 1 (HIV) infection. *Annals of Internal Medicine* 1990;112:727–737.

16. Volberding PA, Lagakos SW, Koch MA et al: Zidovudine in asymptomatic human immunodeficiency virus infection: A controlled trial in persons with fewer than 500 CD4-positive cells per cubic millimeter. *New England Journal of Medicine* 1990;322:941–949.

17. Sarti GM: Aerosolized pentamidine in HIV. *Postgraduate Medicine* 1989;86:54–69.

18. Harvey AM, Johns RJ, McKusick VA, Owens AH, Ross RS: *The Principles and Practice of Medicine.* Norwalk CT, Appleton and Lange, 1988.

19. Davis JH, Foster RS, Gamelli, RL: *Essentials of Clinical Surgery.* St Louis, Mosby Yearbook, 1991.

20. James EC, Corry RJ, Perry JF (eds): *Principles of Basic Surgical Practice*. Philadelphia, Hanley & Belfus, 1987.

21. Liechty RD, Soper RT: *Fundamentals of Surgery*. St Louis, CV Mosby Co, 1989.

22. Ravel R: *Clinical Laboratory Medicine: Clinical Application of Laboratory Data*. Chicago, Year Book Medical Publishers, 1989.

23. Sabiston DC: *Essentials of Surgery*. Philadelphia, WB Saunders, 1987.

24. Silen, W: *Cope's Early Diagnosis of the Acute Abdomen*. New York, Oxford University Press, 1991.

25. Avery ME, First LR (ed): *Pediatric Medicine*. Baltimore, Williams and Wilkins, 1989.

26. Behrman RE, Vaughn VC (ed): *Nelson's Textbook of Pediatrics*, ed 13. Philadelphia, WB Saunders, 1987.

27. Bluestone CD, Klein JO: *Otitis Media in Infants and Children*. Philadelphia, WB Saunders, 1988.

28. Crapo JD, Hamilton MA, Edgman S: *Medicine and Pediatrics in One Book*. Philadelphia, Hanley and Belfus, 1988.

29. Daeschner CW (ed): *Pediatrics, An Approach to Independent Learning*. New York, John Wiley and Sons, 1983.

30. Dershewitz RA (ed): *Ambulatory Pediatric Care*. Philadelphia, JB Lippincott, 1988.

31. Gracey M, Falkner F (ed): *Nutritional Needs and Assessment of Normal Growth*. New York, Raven Press, 1985.

32. Moffet HL: *Pediatric Infectious Diseases, A Problem-Oriented Approach*. JB Lippincott, Philadelphia, 1975.

33. Wood SL, White GL, Murdock RT: Advances in pediatric immunizations. *Physician Assistant* 1988;12[5]:22–48.

34. Reference #34 has been deleted.

35. Woodward GA, Bolte RG: Children riding in the back of pickup trucks: A neglected safety issue. *Pediatrics* 1990;86:683–691

36. Turner TL, Douglas J, Cockburn F: *Craig's Care of the Newly Born Infant,* ed 8. New York, Churchill Livingstone, 1988.

37. Colloton M: Investigating failure to thrive. *Journal of the American Academy of Physician Assistants* 1989;2:359–367.

38. *1990 Physician's Desk Reference,* ed 44. Information on Lotrisone Cream. Oradell NJ, Medical Economics Co, 1990.

39. Brandes EB, Dillard RA: *A Compendium of Drugs and Dosages Most Frequently Used in Pediatric Practice.* Galveston, TX, University of Texas Medical Branch, 1982.

40. Taylor-Watts KT, Starke JR: Tuberculosis in children: A guide to diagnosis, treatment and prevention. *Physician Assistant* 1989;13[3]:29–48.

41. Wyngaarden JB, Smith LH (eds): *Cecil Textbook of Medicine,* ed 18. Philadelphia, WB Saunders, 1988.

42. Harvey AM, Johns RJ, McKusick VA, Owens AH, Ross RS: *The Principles and Practice of Medicine.* Norwalk, CT, Appleton and Lange, 1988.

43. Zalis EG, Connover MH: *Understanding Electrocardiography.* St Louis, Mosby, 1976.

44. Domonokos AN (ed): *Andrew's Diseases of the Skin,* ed 6. Philadelphia, WB Saunders, 1990.

45. Lookingbill DP, Marks JG: *Principles of Dermatology.* Philadelphia, WB Saunders, 1986.

46. Arndt KA: *Manual of Dermatologic Therapeutics,* ed 2. Boston, Little, Brown and Co, 1978.

47. Stein J (ed): *Internal Medicine,* ed 3. Boston. Little, Brown, 1990.

48. Pernoll ML, Benson RC (eds): *Current Obstetric and Gynecologic Diagnosis and Treatment,* ed 6. Norwalk CT, Appleton and Lange, 1987.

49. Dunniho DR: *Fundamentals of Gynecology and Obstetrics.* Philadelphia, JB Lippincott, 1990.

50. Clark-Pearson MD, Dawood MD: *Green's Gynecology: Essentials of Clinical Practice.* Boston, Little, Brown and Co, 1990.

51. U.S. Preventive Services Task Force: *Guide to Clinical Preventive Services.* Baltimore, Williams and Wilkins, 1989.

52. Kane W: *Healthy Living: An Active Approach to Wellness.* Indianapolis, Bobbs-Merrill Educational Publishing, 1985.

53. Bunker JF, Shelton SR, Parcell GS: Health promotion and disease prevention: Roles and strategies for physician assistants. *Physician Assistant* 1987;11:86–96.

54. Physician Associate Program, Emory University School of Medicine: *The Physician Assistant's Guide to Health Promotion and Disease Prevention.* Atlanta, Emory University, 1986.

55. Berkow R et al (eds): *Merck Manual,* ed 15. Rahway, NJ, Merck Sharp & Dohme Research Laboratories, 1987.

56. Braunwald E et al (eds): *Harrison's Principles of Internal Medicine,* ed 11. New York, McGraw-Hill, 1987.

57. Hathaway W et al (eds): *Current Pediatric Diagnosis and Treatment,* ed 10. Norwalk, CT, Appleton and Lange, 1991.

58. Ho MT, Saunders CE (eds): *Current Emergency Diagnosis and Treatment,* ed 3. Norwalk, CT, Appleton and Lange, 1990.

59. Katsung B (ed): *Basic and Clinical Pharmacology,* ed 4. Norwalk, CT, Appleton and Lange, 1989.

60. Pernoll M (ed): *Current Obstetric & Gynecology Diagnosis and Treatment,* ed 7. Norwalk, CT, Appleton and Lange, 1991.

61. Schroeder S et al (eds): *Current Medical Diagnosis and Treatment,* ed 28. Norwalk, CT, Appleton and Lange, 1990.

62. Tintinalli J et al (eds): *Emergency Medicine: A Comprehensive Study Guide,* ed 2. New York, McGraw-Hill, 1988.

63. Vaughn D et al (eds): *General Ophthalmology,* ed 12. Norwalk, CT, Appleton and Lange, 1989.

64. Way L et al (ed): *Current Surgical Diagnosis and Treatment,* ed 9. Norwalk, CT, Appleton and Lange, 1991.

65. Noble J: *Textbook of General Medicine and Primary Care.* Boston, Little, Brown and Co, 1987.

66. Greene HL, Glassock RJ, Kelley, MA (eds): *Introduction to Clinical Medicine.* Philadelphia, BC Decker, 1991.

67. Lee WV et al (eds): *Textbook of Otolaryngology and Head and Neck Surgery.* New York, Elsevier, 1989.

68. Liston SL: Lateral pharyngeal diverticula. *Otolaryngology and Head and Neck Surgery* 1985;93:582–585.

69. Green M et al: Upper airway manifestations of primary ciliary dyskinesia. *Journal of Laryngology and Otology* 1985;99:985–991.

70. Marks MD: *Stigmata of Respiratory Tract Allergies.* Kalamazoo, MI, The UpJohn Company, 1977.

71. Gernon WH: Care and management of acute hematoma of the external ear. *Laryngoscope* 1979;87:881–885.

72. Chandler JR: Malignant external otitis. *Laryngoscope* 1968;78:1257–1294.

73. Crabtree JR: Herpes zosteroticus. *Laryngoscope* 1968;78:1853–1878.

74. Shockley WW et al: Frontal sinus fractures: Some problems and some solutions. *Laryngoscope* 1988;98:18–22.

75. Batsakis JG et al: Adenocarcinoma of the nasal and paranasal cavities. *Archives of Otolaryngology* 1963;77:625.

76. McEvoy GK (ed): *American Hospital Formulary Service Drug Information 86.* Bethesda, MD, American Society of Hospital Pharmacists, 1986.

77. Sabiston DC (ed): *Essentials of Surgery.* Philadelphia, WB Saunders, 1987.

78. Shemen LJ: *Malignant Diseases of the Oral Cavity and Salivary Glands.* New York, Elsevier, 1989.

79. Federman DD: Endocrinology. *Scientific American Medicine* 1989;Section 3:9–11.

80. Moore KL: *Essentials of Human Embryology.* Philadelphia, BC Decker, 1988.

81. Schramm VL, Ettron MZ: Nasal polyps in children. *Laryngoscope* 1980;90:1488–1495.

82. Hoffman IN et al (eds): *Hematology Basic Principles and Practices.* New York, Churchill Livingstone, 1991.